Nursing School Bound

A College Guide For Admission Success

By
Pupil2Peer

FROM PLANNING TO ACTION
CONTAINS OVER 600 NURSING PROGRAMS
SUBMISSION TOOLKIT
WRITTEN BY NURSES FOR FUTURE NURSES

WHERE STRATEGY MEETS NURSING

COPYRIGHT

DISCLAIMER

The author and publisher have reviewed all information in this book with resources believed to be reliable and accurate and have made every effort to provide information that is up to date and correct at the time of publication. Despite our best efforts we cannot guarantee that the information contained herein is complete or fully accurate due to the possibility of the discovery of contradictory information in the future and any human error on part of the author, publisher, and all other parties involved in this work. The author, publisher, and all other parties involved in the work disclaim all responsibility from any errors contained within this work and from any results that arise from the use of this information. Readers are encouraged to check all information in this book with institutional guidelines, other sources, and up to date information.

The information contained in this book is provided for general information purposes only and does not constitute medical, legal, or other professional advice on any subject matter. The author or publisher of this book does not accept any responsibility for any loss which may arise from reliance on information contained within this book or on any associated websites or blogs.

DISCOVER
APPLY
ENROLL

CONTENTS

WELCOME

At Pupil2Peer Nursing Consulting LLC, we are transformational leaders, innovators, and industry consultants committed to fostering inclusion in nursing education to achieve health equity. As a Diversity Movement Partner, we break cycles, change narratives, and streamline new entrants to the healthcare workforce.

Contained herein, you'll find information for prospective students, current students, academic partners, and friends. Place the power of selection in your hand; navigate your journey today!

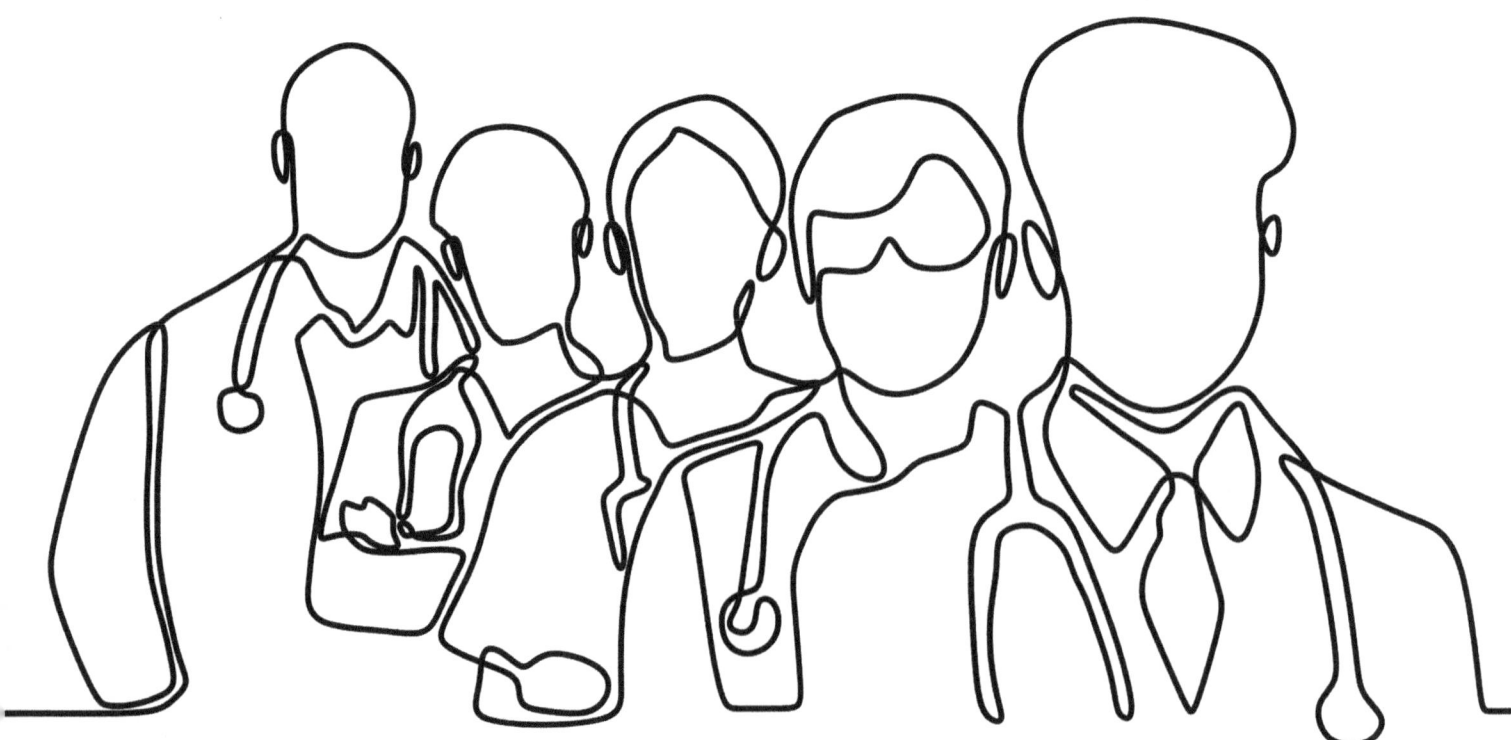

"The path to our destination is not always a straight one.

We go down the wrong road, we get lost, we turn back.

Maybe it doesn't matter which road we embark on.

Maybe what matters is that we embark."

—Barbara Hall

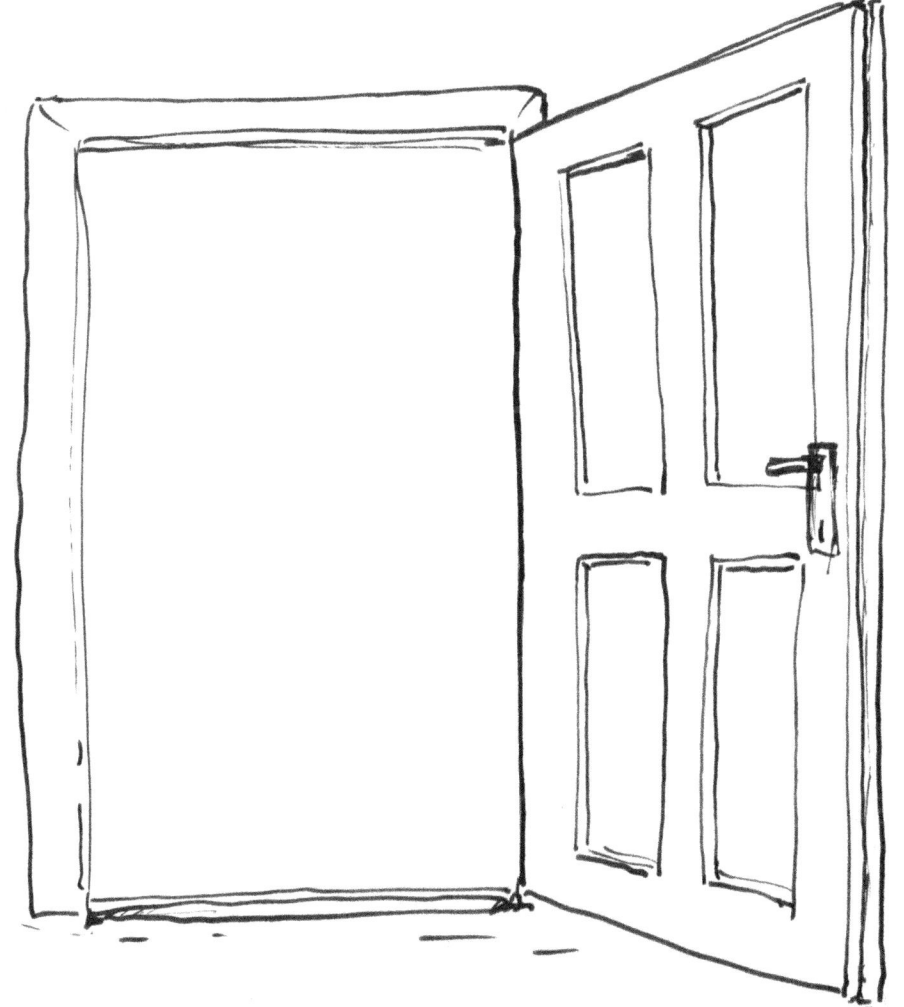

BELIEVE IN
YOURSELF.
THIS BOOK IS
DEDICATED TO **YOU.**

CHAPTER 1

THE FUTURE STATE OF NURSING

SBAR Report

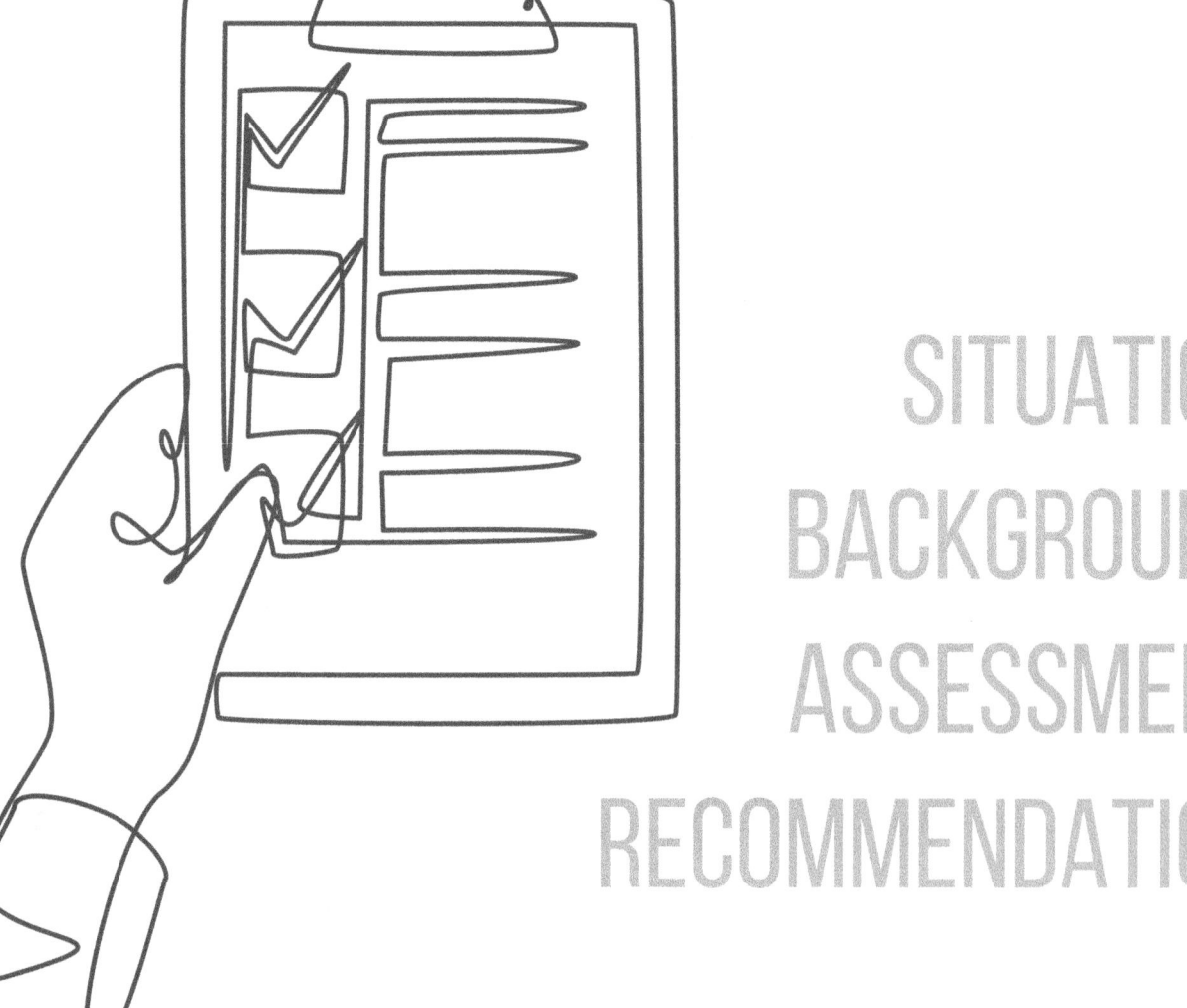

SITUATION

BACKGROUND

ASSESSMENT

RECOMMENDATION

SBAR REPORT

SITUATION:

Covid-19 unveils a crisis within a crisis, the US Nursing Shortage.

BACKGROUND:

As Coronavirus cases skyrocketed and hospitalizations reached unprecedented highs, Covid-19 accelerated changes to a diminishing workforce, exacerbating long-standing nursing shortfalls, highlighting historical inequities, and augmenting what some may perceive as a fractionated healthcare delivery system. In a call-to-action letter to government officials, the American Nurse Association (ANA) delivered a message that made global headlines.

DECLARE NURSING STAFF SHORTAGE A NATIONAL CRISIS.

For years, industry analysts, researchers, and subject matter experts have warned about looming nursing shortages in the United States. In 2010, the Institute of Medicine (IoM) published *The Future of Nursing: Leading Change, Advancing Health*, to assess the current state of nursing, catalyze action, and drive change for the future.

According to the Bureau of Labor Statistics, Registered Nursing (RN) is among the top occupations in job growth through 2029. Putting complex numbers to this, analysts expect the nursing workforce to grow from 3 million in 2019 to 3.3 million in 2029, an increase of 221,900 or 7%. The Bureau also projects 175,900 openings for RNs each year through 2029, when nurse retirements and workforce exits are factored into the number of nurses needed in the US.

Add a global pandemic, and that shortage is here now.

ASSESSMENT:

Every day, thousands transition into the population segment of adults aged 65 and up. This growing quartile has different demographics and needs, causing health systems to question their adaptability and sustainability. Compounding the problem is that nursing schools across the country are in a race against time.

SUPPLY VS. DEMAND.

Notably, in 2019-2020 the American Association of Colleges of Nursing (AACN) reported that US nursing schools turned away 80,407 qualified applicants from baccalaureate and graduate nursing programs due to insufficient faculty, clinical sites, classroom space, clinical preceptors, and budget constraints.

With entrance to practice barriers and experience-complexity gaps at their heels, industry leaders have found themselves in an unprecedented flux as they battle pandemic hardships and implement workforce recovery.

THE PROBLEM – AND THE SOLUTION – STARTS AT THE TOP.

To help prioritize priorities, stakeholders such as the National Council of State Boards of Nursing (NCSBN), the world leader in nursing regulatory knowledge, deep-dived into where the industry is going and aid in uncovering proven solutions through analytics and best practices. Researchers predict that the decade ahead will demand a more robust, more diversified nursing workforce prepared to provide care, promote health and well-being among nurses, individuals, and communities, and address the systemic inequities fueled by wide and persistent health disparities.

In collaborative partnerships, NCSBN conducts the only national-level survey focused on the US nursing workforce every two years. Data collected between February 19, 2020, and June 30, 2020, through a randomized study of 157,459 Registered Nurses (RNs) and 172,045 Licensed Practical/Vocational Nurses (LPN/VNs) revealed the following:

- Nearly 81% of RNs reported being White/Caucasian.
- RNs who reported being Asian accounted for 7.2% of the workforce, representing the largest non-Caucasian racial group in the RN workforce.
- Black/African American RNs increased from 6.0 % in 2013 to 6.7 % in 2020.
- 19.2% of RN respondents self-reported as a minority, including "other" and "two or more races."
- Males accounted for 9.4% of the RN workforce.
- The median age of RNs was found to be 52 years old.
- LPN/VNs were more racially diverse than their RN counterparts, with approximately 29% of LPN/VNs identifying as racial minorities

CAN WE CLOSE THE GAP?

RECOMMENDATIONS:

CREATE A DIVERSE ENTRY-LEVEL PIPELINE.

The committee of *The Future of Nursing 2020-2030: Charting a Path to Health Equity* said it best, **"Efforts to recruit and educate prospective nurses to serve a diverse population and advance health equity will be fruitless unless accompanied by efforts to acknowledge and dismantle racism within nursing education and nursing practice."**

4

With thought-provoking empathy, they vividly described the "isolation" and "loss of self" that many minority students face in their pursuit of nursing, calling upon institutions to critically examine their own cultures. In solidarity, Pupil2Peer advocates maintaining nursing excellence with a constant focus on innovation, addressing pipeline deficiencies, retention pain points, and structural barriers to nursing practice. We challenge societal norms and employ "good trouble."

Seeking beyond band-aid solutions, we recommend initiatives such as streamlining integrated nursing pathways, providing academic, financial support, and transitional mentorship to underserved and minority students, new graduate preparedness, and working with community partners as vessels of belonging. While also increasing the availability and visibility of minority faculty and organizational leadership, steering the creation of workplace inclusion and diversity to achieve health equity for all.

BE THE CHANGE.

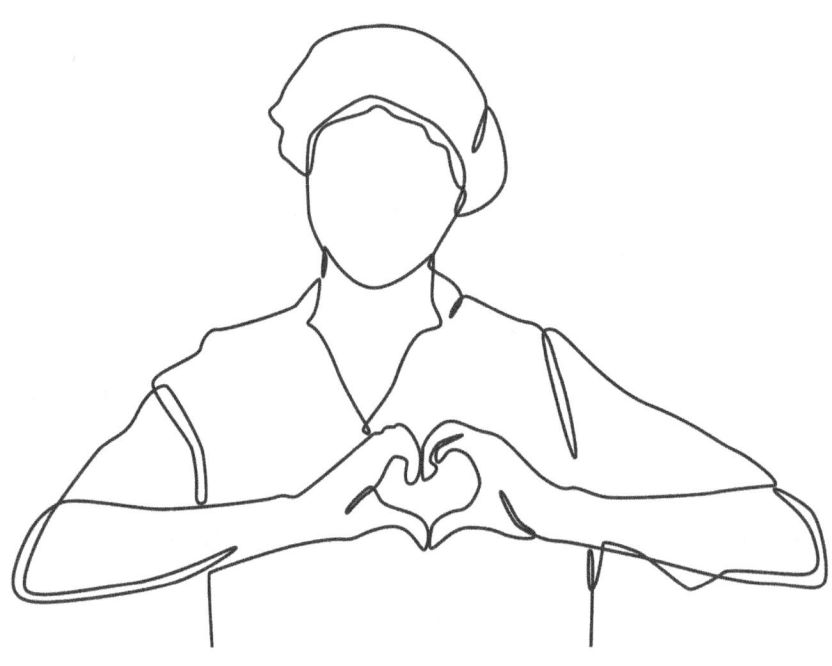

"ONCE YOU FIND YOUR WHY, YOU WILL BE ABLE TO FIND YOUR WAY. WHY IS YOUR PURPOSE. WAY IS YOUR PATH."

– JOHN MAXWELL

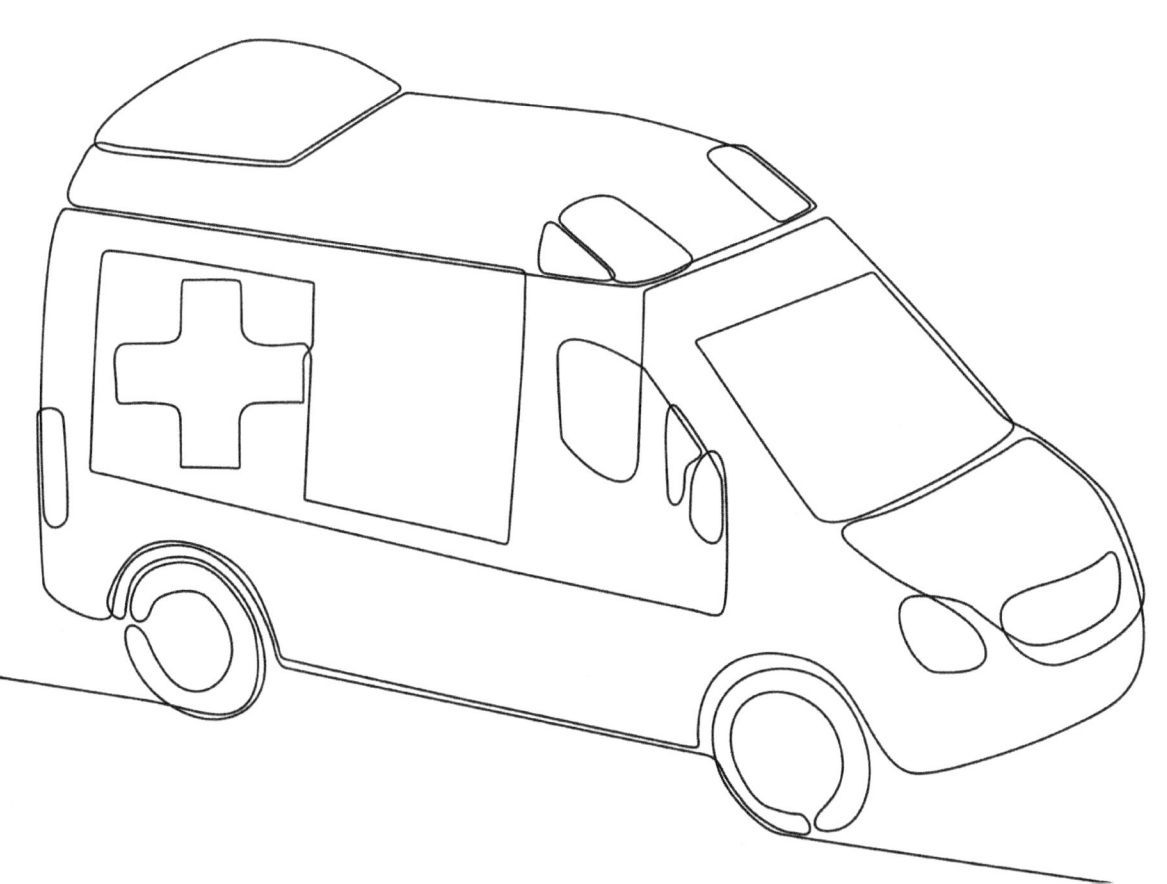

CHAPTER 2
PATHWAYS TO A BSN DEGREE

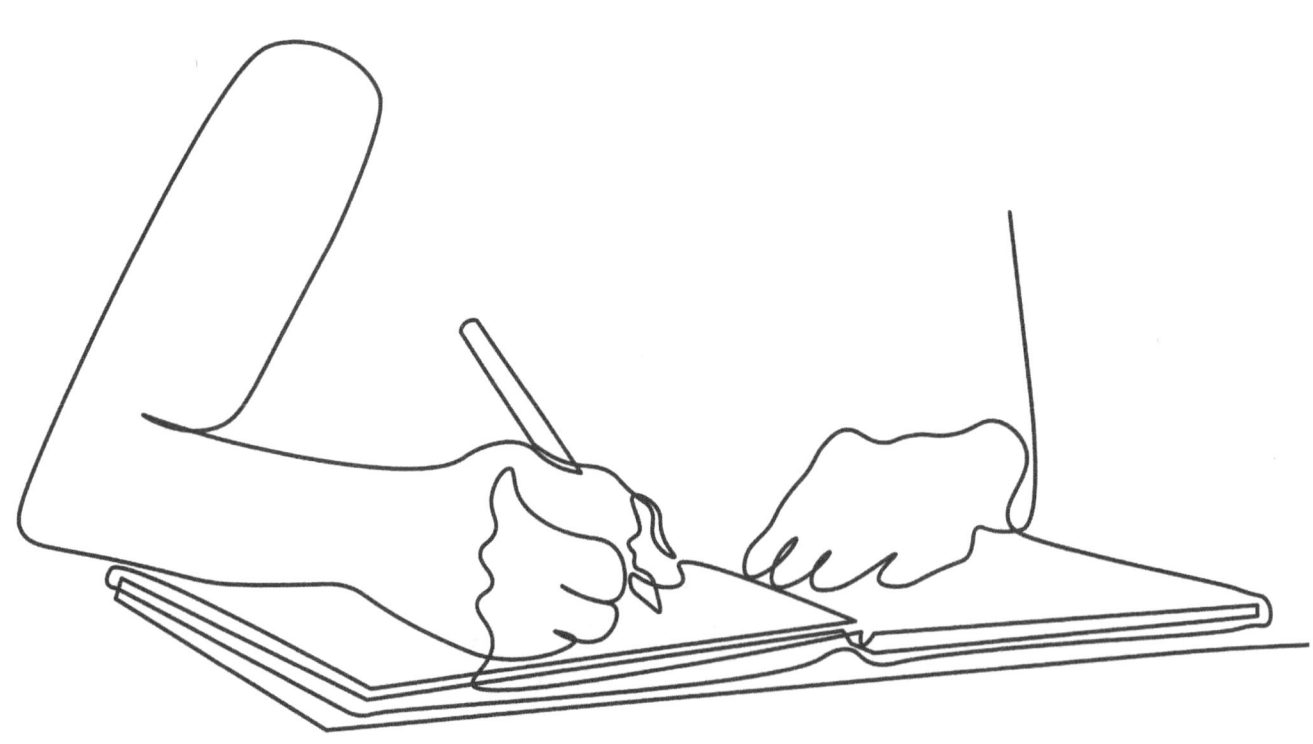

There is often more than one way to peel an orange. Well, pupils, that also applies to nursing. Universities and colleges are large scaling their program efforts for solutions that match the severe gravity of the shortage.

What kind of future career are you looking for? Review the following academic pathways to find the right starting point for you!

LICENSED PRACTICAL NURSE/LICENSED VOCATIONAL NURSE (LVN/LPN)

ASSOCIATE DEGREE IN NURSING (ADN)

BACHELOR OF SCIENCE IN NURSING (BSN)

ACCELERATED BACHELOR OF SCIENCE IN NURSING (ABSN)

LICENSED PRACTICAL NURSE/ LICENSED VOCATIONAL NURSE (LVN/LPN)

A program that awards a diploma or certificate of completion as an LPN/LVN

COURSE LENGTH

9 to 12 months

EXPECTED SALARY

$29k–$50k

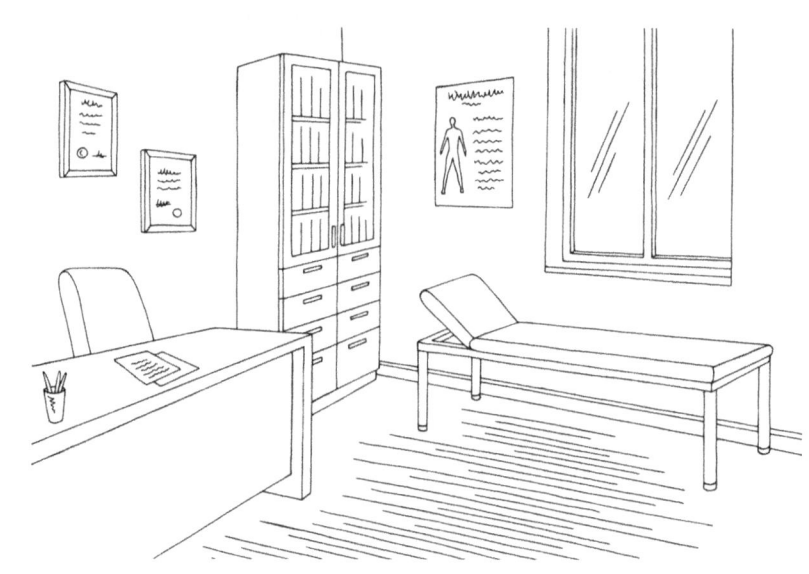

PATIENT CARE

Under the supervision of an RN or primary care provider, your duties will include monitoring patients, administering medication, collecting data, and performing other hands-on tasks.

WHERE YOU'LL WORK

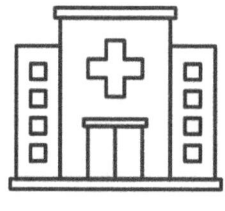 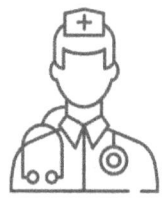 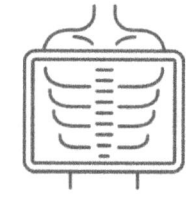 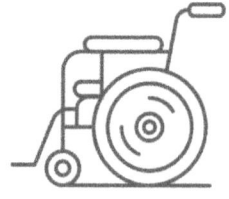

| HOSPITALS | DOCTOR'S OFFICES | OUTPATIENT CARE CENTERS | NURSING HOMES |

LICENSURE EXAM

NCLEX-PN

Before practicing, you must pass this standardized exam set by the Board of Nursing in every state. It's designed to ensure you're ready to work as an entry-level nurse.

CAREER LADDER

One of the best things about being a nurse is that? You'll never stop learning. You'll have opportunities to grow from the day you start your career.

CONTINUE YOUR EDUCATION

Most places you'll work will offer courses that keep your skills sharp and your knowledge up to date.

GET AN ADN/ASN

An Associate's Degree in Nursing (ADN) or Associate of Science in Nursing (ASN) is the next step in nursing.

GET A BSN

A Bachelor of Science in Nursing (BSN) will earn you more responsibilities and opportunities.

Source: LPN/LVN Certificate | Johnson & Johnson Nursing (jnj.com

ASSOCIATE DEGREE IN NURSING (ADN)

A program that requires at least two academic years of full-time equivalent coursework and awards an associate degree in nursing.

COURSE LENGTH

24 months

EXPECTED SALARY

$54k–$88k

PATIENT CARE

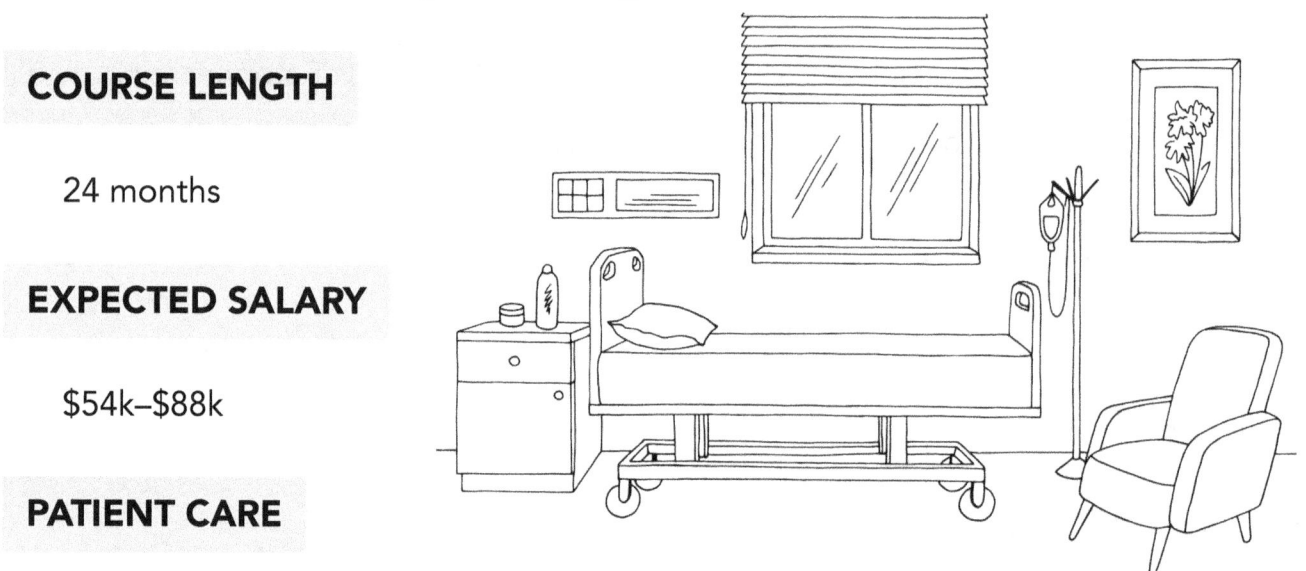

You'll get experience in many different specialties while working with doctors and other Registered Nurses in hospitals, clinics, and healthcare facilities.

WHERE YOU'LL WORK

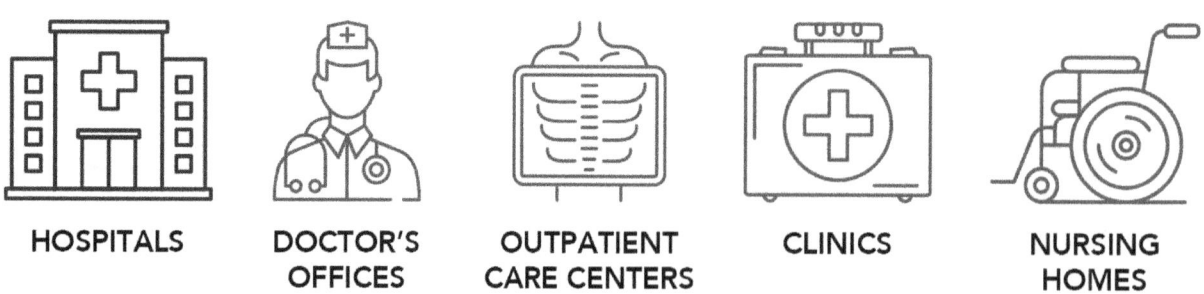

HOSPITALS   DOCTOR'S OFFICES   OUTPATIENT CARE CENTERS   CLINICS   NURSING HOMES

LICENSURE EXAM

NCLEX-RN

Before you can start practicing, you must pass this standardized exam set by the Board of Nursing in every state. It's designed to ensure you're ready to work as a Registered Nurse.

CAREER LADDER

One of the best things about being a nurse is that? You'll never stop learning. You'll have opportunities to grow from the day you start your career.

CONTINUE YOUR EDUCATION

Most places you'll work will offer courses that keep your skills sharp and your knowledge up to date.

GET A BSN

A Bachelor of Science in Nursing (BSN) will earn you more responsibilities and opportunities.

Source: ADN Nursing | Johnson & Johnson Nursing (jnj.com)

BACHELOR OF SCIENCE IN NURSING (BSN)

Admits students with no previous nursing education and awards a baccalaureate nursing degree.

COURSE LENGTH

4 years

AVERAGE ANNUAL SALARY

$57k–$130k

WHAT YOU'LL DO

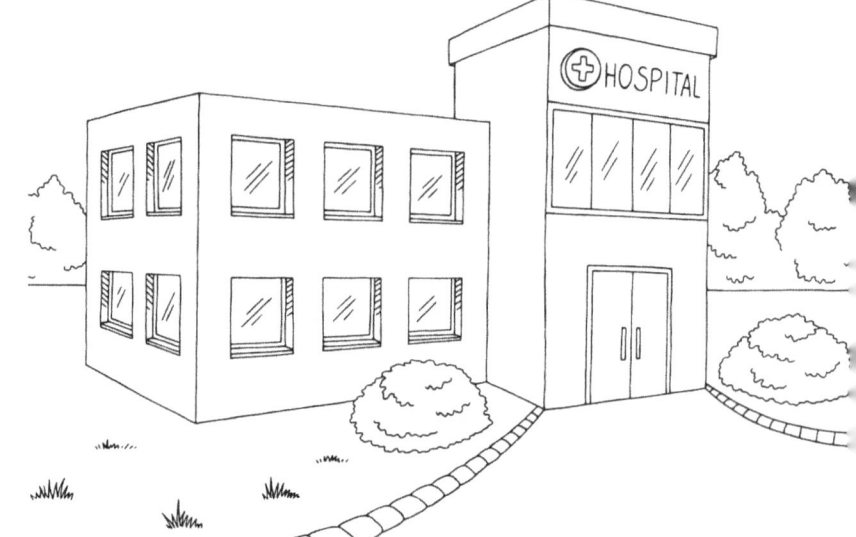

Nurses with a BSN are in demand. You'll have a choice of where you want to work and what you'd like to specialize in when you enter the field.

MANAGERIAL DUTIES

With a BSN, you'll be prepped for a leadership role and gradually take on more responsibilities, such as developing treatment plans, educating patients, and supervising other nurses

PATIENT CARE

You'll work with doctors and other Registered Nurses, administering medications and injections and caring for patients and their families.

WHERE YOU'LL WORK

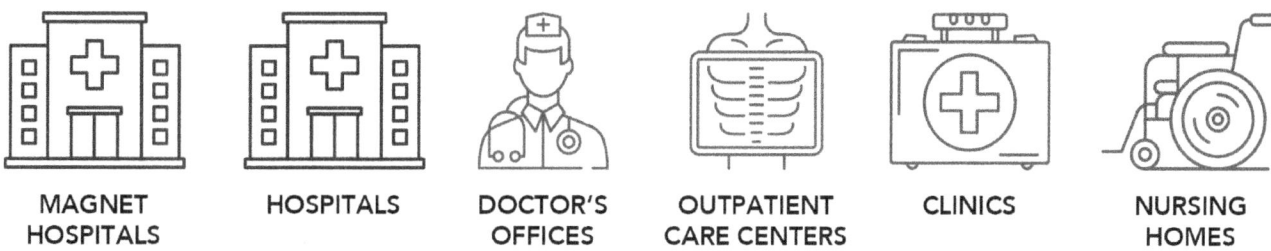

MAGNET HOSPITALS   HOSPITALS   DOCTOR'S OFFICES   OUTPATIENT CARE CENTERS   CLINICS   NURSING HOMES

LICENSURE EXAM

NCLEX-RN

Before you can start practicing, you must pass this standardized exam set by the Board of Nursing in every state. It's designed to ensure you're ready to work as a Registered Nurse.

DID YOU KNOW

NURSES WITH A BSN ARE ELIGIBLE FOR 88% OF NURSING POSITIONS.

Source: https://nursejournal.org/bsn-degree/top-9-advantages-of-a-bsn-degree
Source: BSN Degree | Johnson & Johnson Nursing (jnj.com)

ACCELERATED BACHELOR OF SCIENCE IN NURSING (ABSN)

Admits students with a non-nursing baccalaureate degree and awards a baccalaureate nursing degree.

COURSE LENGTH

11 - 18 months

AVERAGE ANNUAL SALARY

$57k–$130k

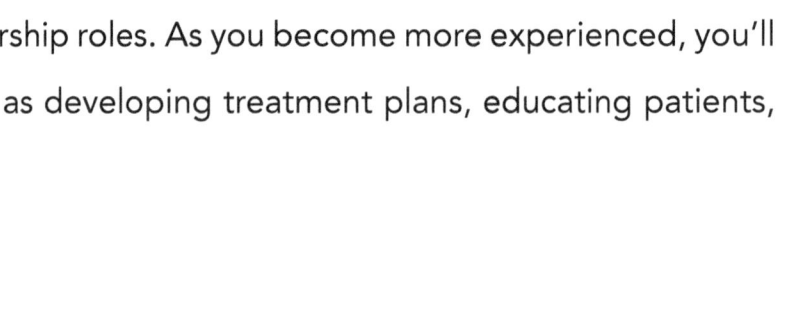

WHAT YOU'LL DO

With an ABSN, you'll have many job opportunities and the chance to grow your career.

MANAGERIAL DUTIES

You'll be trained to take on leadership roles. As you become more experienced, you'll be given more responsibilities, such as developing treatment plans, educating patients, and supervising other nurses.

PATIENT CARE

You'll work with doctors and other Registered Nurses, administering medication and injections and caring for patients and their families.

WHERE YOU'LL WORK

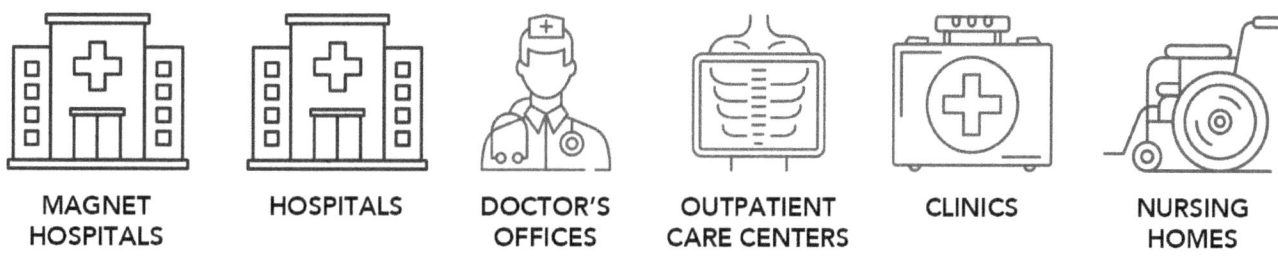

| MAGNET HOSPITALS | HOSPITALS | DOCTOR'S OFFICES | OUTPATIENT CARE CENTERS | CLINICS | NURSING HOMES |

LICENSURE EXAM

NCLEX-RN

Before you can start practicing, you must pass this standardized exam set by the Board of Nursing in every state. It's designed to ensure you're ready to work as a Registered Nurse.

DID YOU KNOW

AN ACCELERATED BACHELOR OF SCIENCE IN NURSING (ABSN) IS THE FAST TRACK TO A NURSING CAREER IF YOU HAVE A DEGREE IN ANOTHER FIELD.

Source: ABSN Degree | Johnson & Johnson Nursing (jnj.com)

"TO SOAR TOWARD WHAT'S POSSIBLE, YOU MUST LEAVE BEHIND WHAT'S COMFORTABLE."

– CICELY TYSON

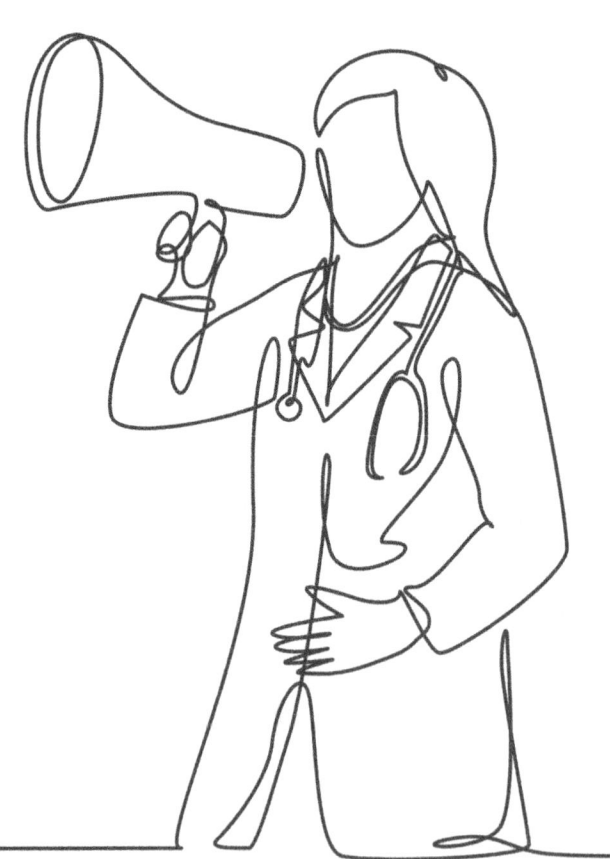

CHAPTER 3
CHOOSE YOUR STARTING POINT

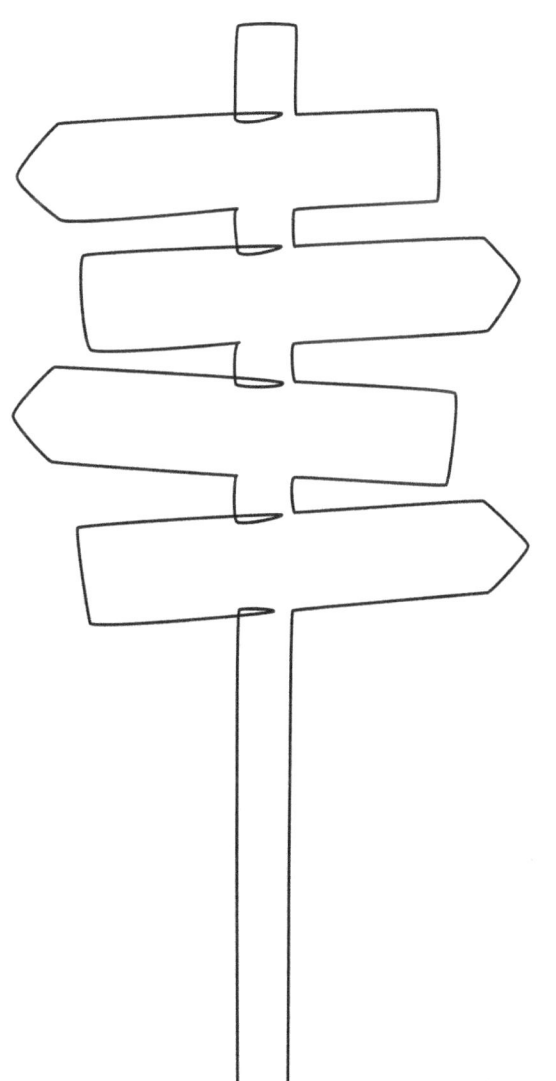

THERE ARE MANY DIFFERENT PATHWAYS TO A NURSING CAREER.

CHOOSE A STARTING POINT TO GET A PERSONALIZED GUIDE OF THE STEPS YOU'LL NEED TO TAKE.

STARTING WITHOUT HEALTHCARE EXPERIENCE

STARTING WITH HEALTHCARE EXPERIENCE

STARTING WITHOUT HEALTHCARE EXPERIENCE

Graduating from high school or already having a degree and wanting to pursue a new career in nursing? Start here.

HIGH SCHOOL STUDENT

FIRST-TIME GRADUATE

COLLEGE GRADUATE

HIGH SCHOOL STUDENT

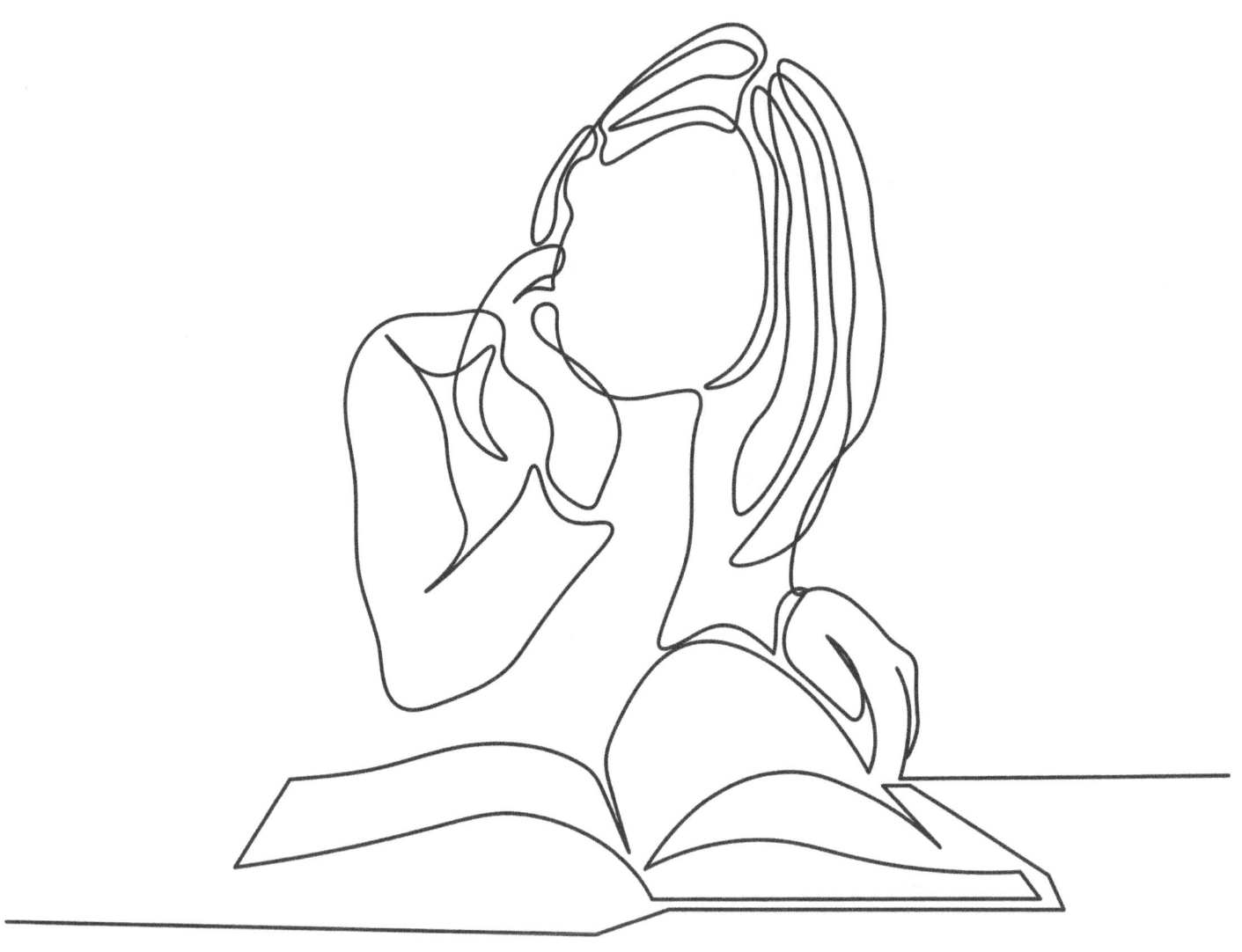

ARE YOU GRADUATING FROM HIGH SCHOOL AND WANTING TO PURSUE A NEW CAREER IN NURSING?

STEP 1: CHOOSE A PROGRAM

The best foundation for a nursing career is a Bachelor of Science in Nursing (BSN). It'll give you many choices when you start working and make it easy to advance your nursing career if you want to.

STEP 2: FIND A SCHOOL AND APPLY

Once you've chosen a program, you'll pick a school. There are over 1,800 nursing schools in the US.

STEP 3: PREPARE TO ENTER THE FIELD

After earning a degree, you must pass the NCLEX-RN, a standardized exam set by the Board of Nursing in each state. It qualifies you to practice as a licensed Registered Nurse.

FIRST-TIME GRADUATE

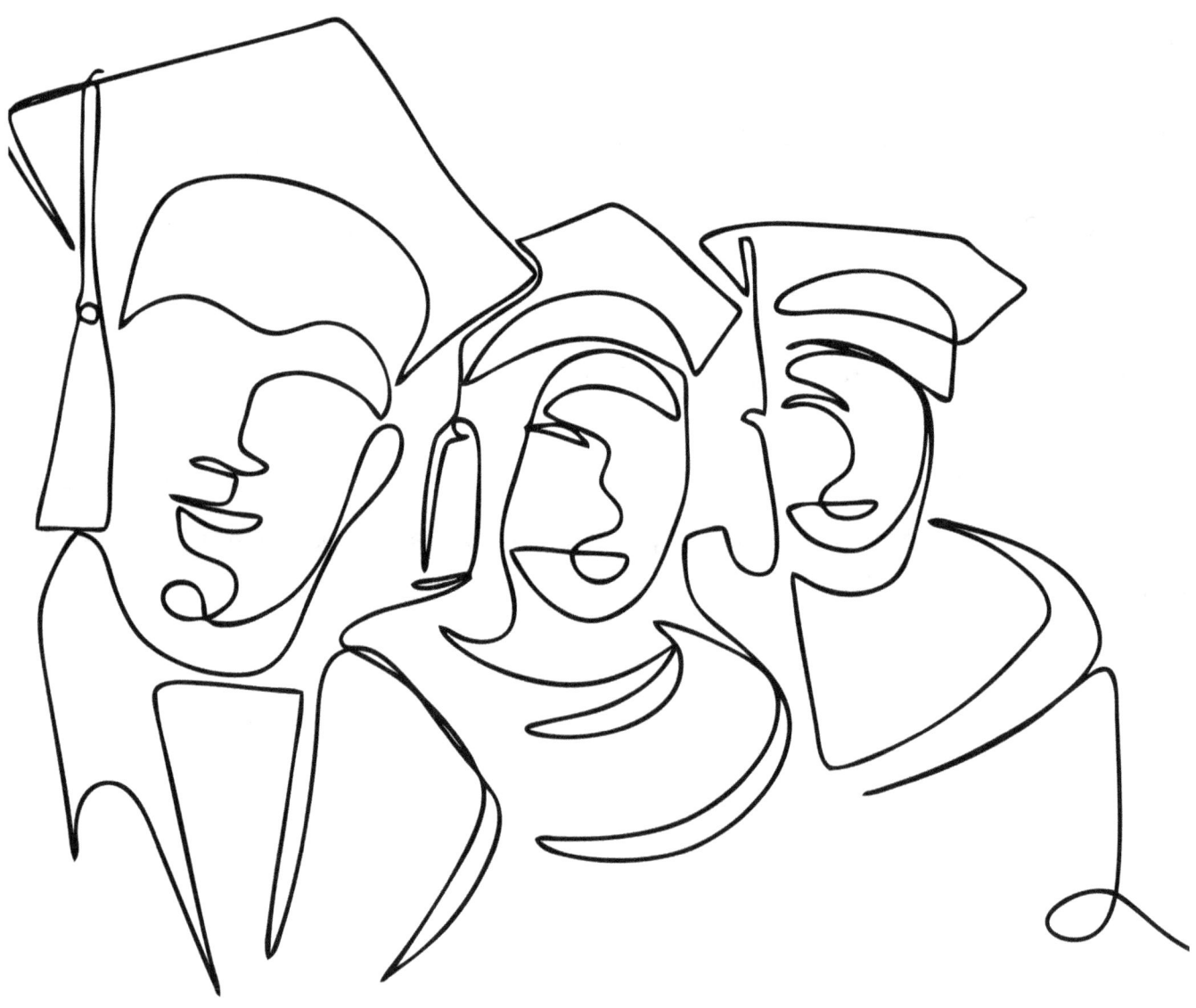

ARE YOU PURSUING YOUR FIRST DEGREE AND LOOKING FOR GROWTH OPPORTUNITIES IN NURSING?

STEP 1: CHOOSE A PROGRAM

You first have to get a degree, and a Bachelor of Science in Nursing (BSN) is the best way to go. It's a stepping-stone to many opportunities and will set you up for an advanced career in nursing.

STEP 2: FIND A SCHOOL AND APPLY

Once you've chosen a program, you'll pick a school. There are over 1,800 nursing schools in the US.

STEP 3: PREPARE TO ENTER THE FIELD

After earning a degree, you must pass the NCLEX-RN, a standardized exam set by the Board of Nursing in each state. It qualifies you to practice as a licensed Registered Nurse.

COLLEGE GRADUATE

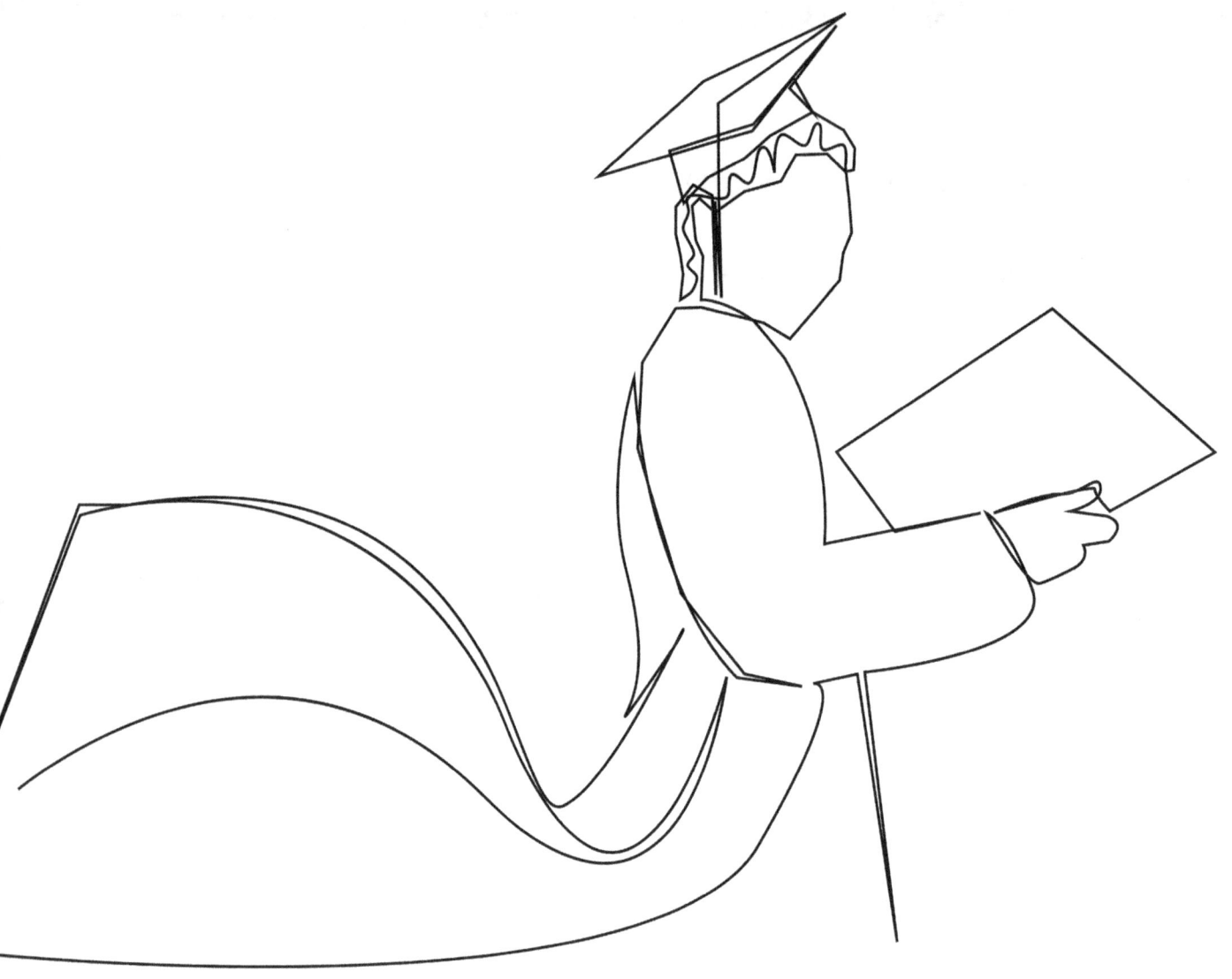

ARE YOU A COLLEGE GRADUATE WITH THE READINESS TO BEGIN A NEW CAREER IN THE 21ST CENTURY AS A BSN?

STEP 1: CHOOSE A PROGRAM

If you've already earned a degree in another field, you can fast-track your nursing career by studying for an Accelerated Bachelor of Science in Nursing (ABSN). This degree will give you many choices and opportunities as a nurse.

STEP 2: FIND A SCHOOL AND APPLY

Once you've chosen a program, you'll pick a school. There are over 1,800 nursing schools in the US.

STEP 3: PREPARE TO ENTER THE FIELD

After earning a degree, you must pass the NCLEX-RN, a standardized exam set by the Board of Nursing in each state. It qualifies you to practice as a licensed Registered Nurse.

STARTING WITH HEALTHCARE EXPERIENCE

Do you already have some medical experience? Start here if you've worked in healthcare before.

CORPSMAN

NURSE OUTSIDE OF NORTH AMERICA

NURSE IN CANADA OR MEXICO

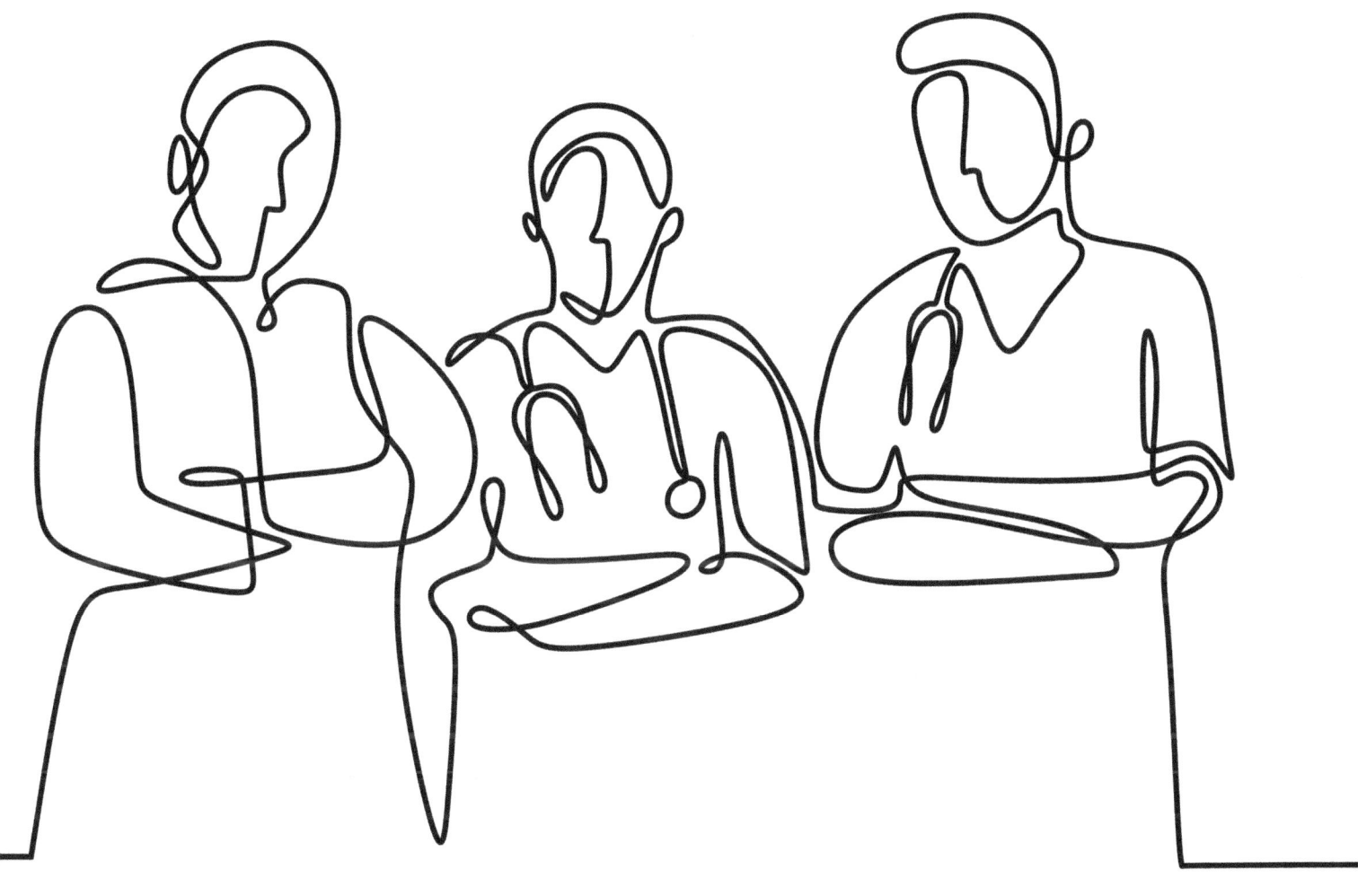

DO YOU WISH TO TRANSITION FROM A HEALTHCARE ROLE IN THE MILITARY TO A CIVILIAN ROLE AS A REGISTERED NURSE?

STEP 1: CHOOSE A PROGRAM

Your healthcare experience may qualify you for a bridge program that'll help you become a Registered Nurse without repeating any previous training. First, you'll find a suitable program. It can even be online if you want more flexibility. Bridge programs are shorter, giving you the chance to advance faster.

Examples:

- *Veteran to BSN*
- *VBSN (Veterans' BSN)*
- *Military to BSN*

STEP 2: FIND A SCHOOL AND APPLY

Once you've chosen a program, you'll pick a school. There are over 1,800 nursing schools in the US.

STEP 3: PREPARE TO ENTER THE FIELD

After earning a degree, you must pass the NCLEX-RN, a standardized exam set by the Board of Nursing in each state. It qualifies you to practice as a licensed Registered Nurse.

NURSE OUTSIDE OF NORTH AMERICA

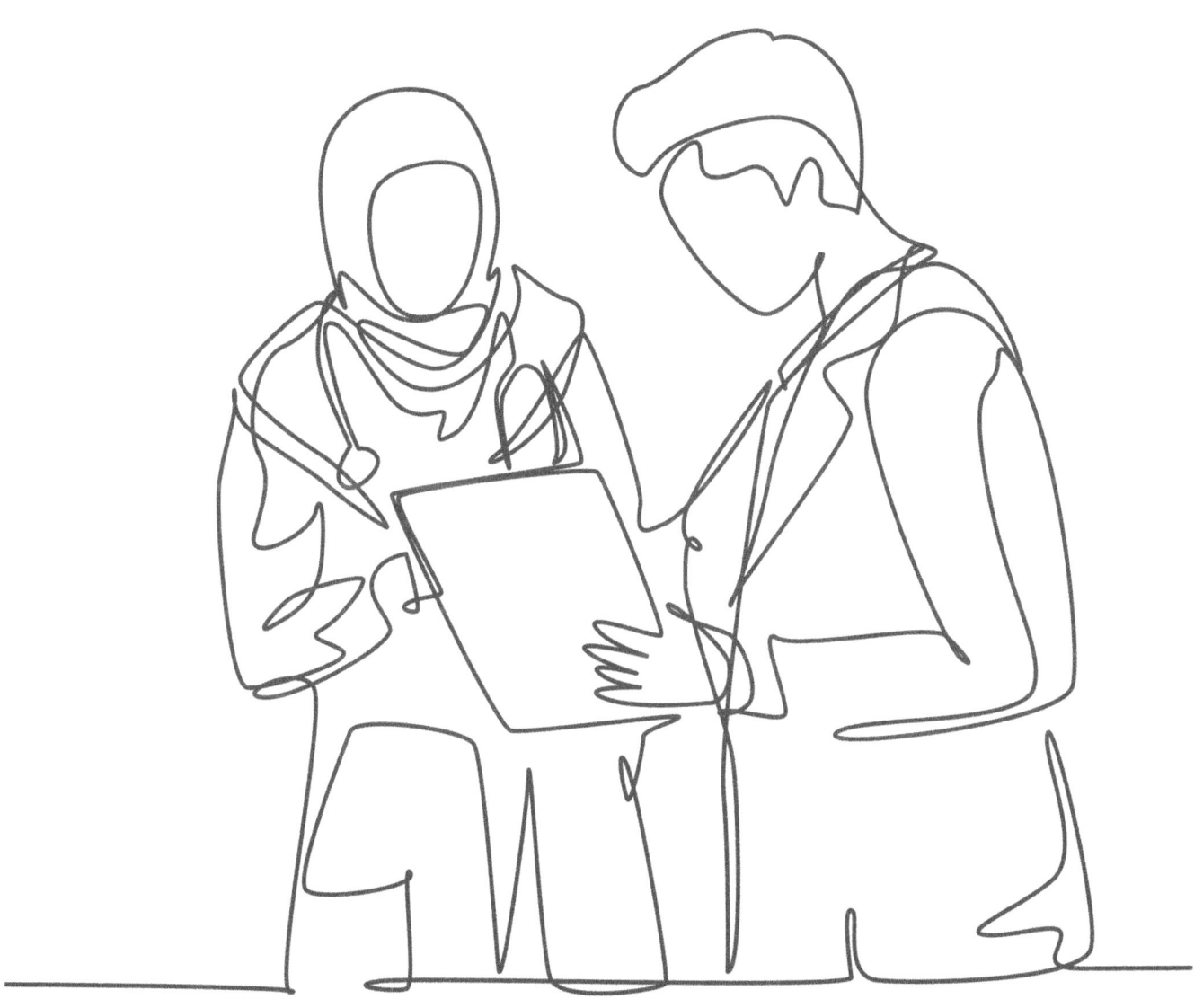

DO YOU HAVE HEALTHCARE EXPERIENCE AS A NURSE OUTSIDE OF NORTH AMERICA AND ARE LOOKING TO WORK IN THE US?

STEP 1

First, you must be a Registered Nurse in your home country. If you are, contact the Commission on Graduates of Foreign Nursing Schools (CGFNS) to see if you're qualified to work in the US.

STEP 2

Once you've passed the prescreening, you must apply to the state where you'd like to work's Board of Nursing and pass the NCLEX-RN to get a Registered Nurse license. It may include an English language proficiency test.

STEP 3

The next step is to find a suitable position through a nursing recruitment agency or US-based employer.

STEP 4

Lastly, you need to get a nonimmigrant visa that will allow you to work in the US. When you've worked for a certain number of years, you can be sponsored for a Green Card by a US employer.

NURSE IN CANADA OR MEXICO

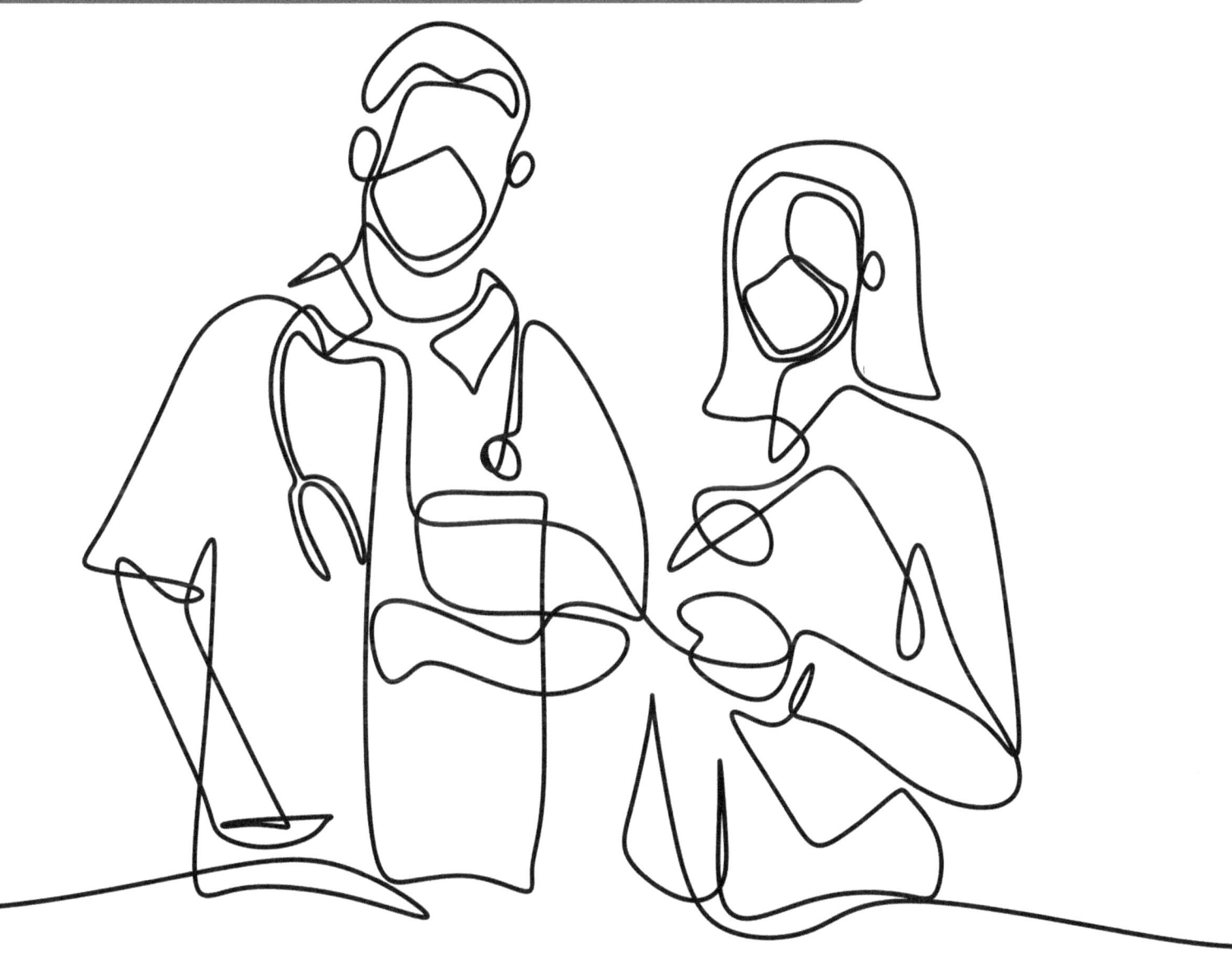

DO YOU HAVE HEALTHCARE EXPERIENCE AS A NURSE IN CANADA OR MEXICO AND ARE LOOKING TO WORK IN THE US?

STEP 1

First, you must be a citizen of Canada or Mexico with a state or provincial license to practice in your home country. You'll need to contact the Commission on Graduates of Foreign Nursing Schools (CGFNS) to see if you qualify.

STEP 2

Once you've passed the prescreening, you must apply to the state where you'd like to work's Board of Nursing and pass the NCLEX-RN to get a Registered Nurse license. It may include an English language proficiency test.

STEP 3

The next step is to find a suitable position through a nursing recruitment agency or US-based employer.

STEP 4

Lastly, you need to get a Trade National Visa (TN) that will allow you to work in the US. The TN visa is only available to citizens from Canada and Mexico. When you've worked for a certain number of years, you can be sponsored for a Green Card by a US employer.

"YOU WERE BORN TO WIN, BUT TO BE A WINNER, YOU MUST PLAN TO WIN, PREPARE TO WIN, AND EXPECT TO WIN."

- ZIG ZIGLAR

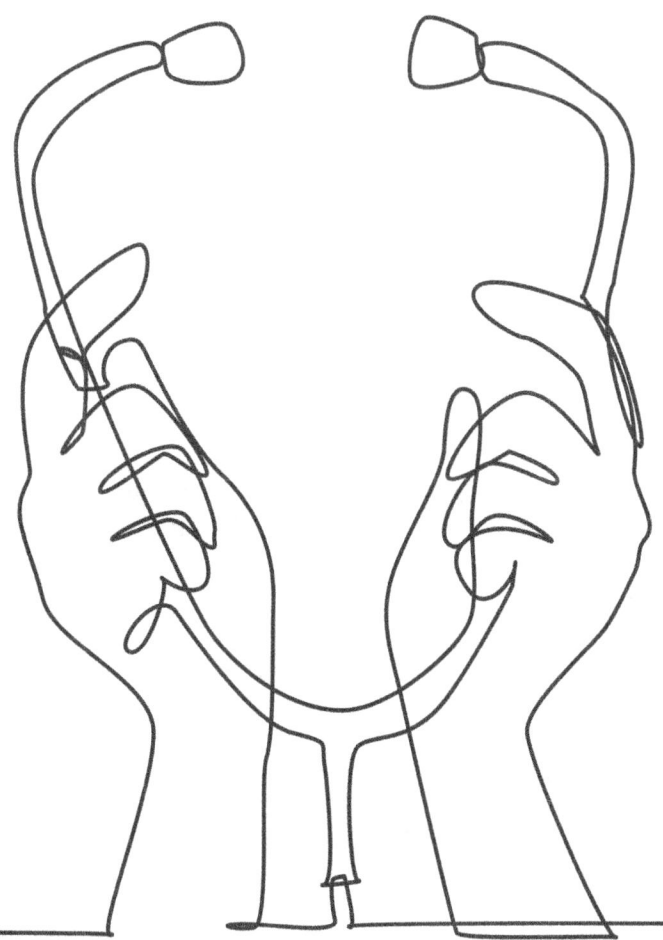

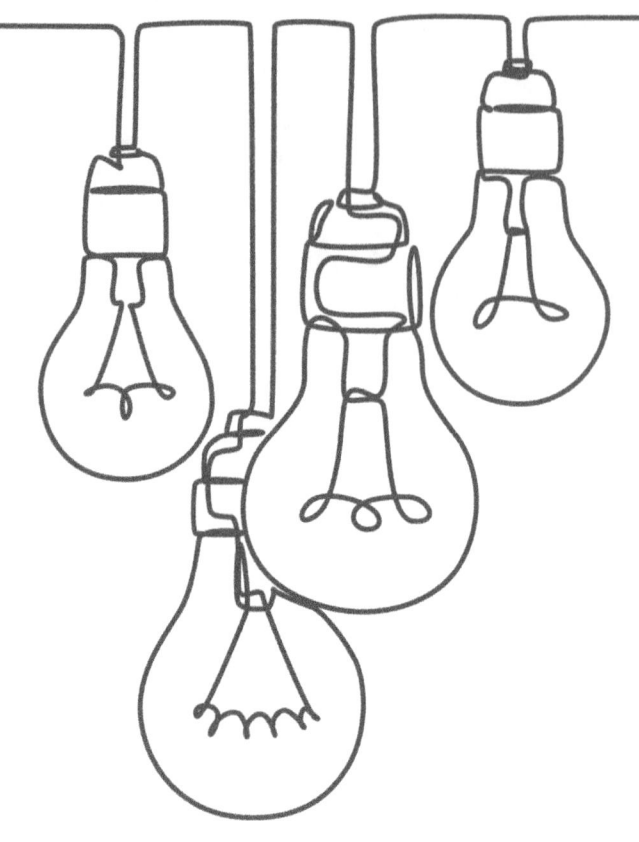

CHAPTER 4

SIX FACTORS TO CONSIDER WHEN SELECTING A NURSING SCHOOL

Imagine buying your first car. You're cost-conscious, quality-driven, evaluating brand and model reputation, and last but not least, you're comparing lifestyle congruence. What you discovered shaped your buying strategy and placed you one step closer behind the wheel.

WE ARE EXERCISING THE POWER OF SELECTION.

Amidst the COVID pandemic, nursing programs have had to make drastic adjustments to market, recruit, and retain prospective students. In an increasingly consumer-driven marketplace, they've learned student preferences, consumer behaviors, and what drives one student to choose one institution over the other.

WHAT STUDENTS NEED: MORE SKIN IN THE GAME.

To determine if your potential school is a "true fit" before you commit, let's explore six factors to consider when selecting a nursing school.

Let's take a deep dive!

DEGREE CHOICE

NATIONAL ACCREDITATION

NCLEX FIRST-TIME PASS RATES

STUDENT-TO-FACULTY RATIO

PROGRAM COST AND FINANCIAL AID AVAILABILITY

JOB PLACEMENT FOLLOWING GRADUATION

#1 DEGREE CHOICE

Considering your timeline and objectives is one way to narrow down the selection. No matter the choice, there is no wrong answer. Whether to pursue an LVN, ADN, or BSN, aligning yourself with a pathway that can channel your passion for helping and serving others is the right degree choice for you.

#2 NATIONAL ACCREDITATION

In two words or less, accreditation is about **quality control**. According to the US Department of Education, accreditation is meant to:

1. Assess the quality of academic programs at institutions of higher education.
2. Create a culture of continuous improvement of academic quality at colleges and universities and stimulate a general raising of standards among educational institutions.
3. Involve faculty and staff comprehensively in institutional evaluation and planning.
4. Establish criteria for professional certification, licensure, and upgrading courses offering such preparation.

In nursing, accreditation aims to ensure that nursing education programs across the United States are parallel in structure and delivery. Thus, it furthers the profession and dramatically enhances nurses› overall quality of care.

WHY IS ACCREDITATION IMPORTANT?

Attending an accredited nursing program allows students to:

- Receive federal and state funding
- Acquire eligible transfer credits

- Pursue graduate nursing endeavors

- Obtain job market competitiveness

It is also essential to highlight the difference between national accreditation and state board approval. State board approval means that the state has approved the program's operation. In most cases, program graduates can sit for licensure or certification exams in that state. At the same time, national accreditation means that the program adheres to common standards of quality set by a US Department of Education-approved agency. Accreditation helps ensure that a nurse educated in Texas and a nurse educated in New Hampshire can perform their duties with the same level of competence.

To help summarize their differences, here's a chart below:

National Accreditation	*State Board Approval*
• Prepares you for licensure and practice • Allows you to sit for the NCLEX exam • Qualifies you for federal and state funding • Enables students to acquire transfer credits or apply coursework to an advanced degree	• Prepares you for licensure and practice • Allows you to sit for the NCLEX exam

ACCREDITING BODIES

Two national organizations that accredit nursing programs include:

The Commission on Collegiate Nursing Education (CCNE)

- CCNE accreditation supports and encourages continuing self-assessment by nursing programs and supports continuing growth and improvement of collegiate, professional education, and nurse residency programs.
- CCNE is the American Association of Colleges of Nursing (AACN) accrediting arm.

The Accreditation Commission for Education in Nursing (ACEN)

- The ACEN is a voluntary, peer-review, self-regulatory process in which non-governmental associations recognize nursing schools or programs that meet or exceed the highest education standards.

HOW DO I KNOW A PROGRAM IS ACCREDITED?

- Each accrediting body maintains a list or database of accredited programs. These are easy to find online and will be the most accurate resource for determining accreditation status.
- An informed consumer is a smart buyer. Checking in on a program's accreditation landscape will make you just that.

#3 NCLEX FIRST-TIME PASS RATES

This is where a program's academic and clinical objectives yield examination success! A high pass rate validates a student's preparedness, but a low pass rate should be considered a huge red flag. Be assertive and ask schools to provide you with their record of examination rates for the past few years.

#4 STUDENT-TO-FACULTY RATIO

The student-to-faculty ratio is a standard metric used to gauge instructional physicality and accessibility to provide an inclusive learning experience for all students. Research has shown that smaller class sizes foster student engagement, interactive learning, and resources for leadership, teaching, mentorship, and scholarship.

#5 PROGRAM COST AND FINANCIAL AID AVAILABILITY

Your future is a financial investment. Your goal should be to get the absolute best education for the least amount of money. Considering the total cost, availability, and accessibility of scholarships, grants, and financial aid when making this critical decision is crucial. Remember, thousands of schools across the country offer nursing degrees. You do not have to go into debt to join our fold.

#6 JOB PLACEMENT FOLLOWING GRADUATION

Partnerships that leverage your educational experience with your career ambitions are professional goals. These programs will house affiliations with renowned hospitals, clinical collaborations, and resources to help you succeed. Harness your full power of networking and inquire about career services.

YOUR FUTURE IS LIMITLESS.

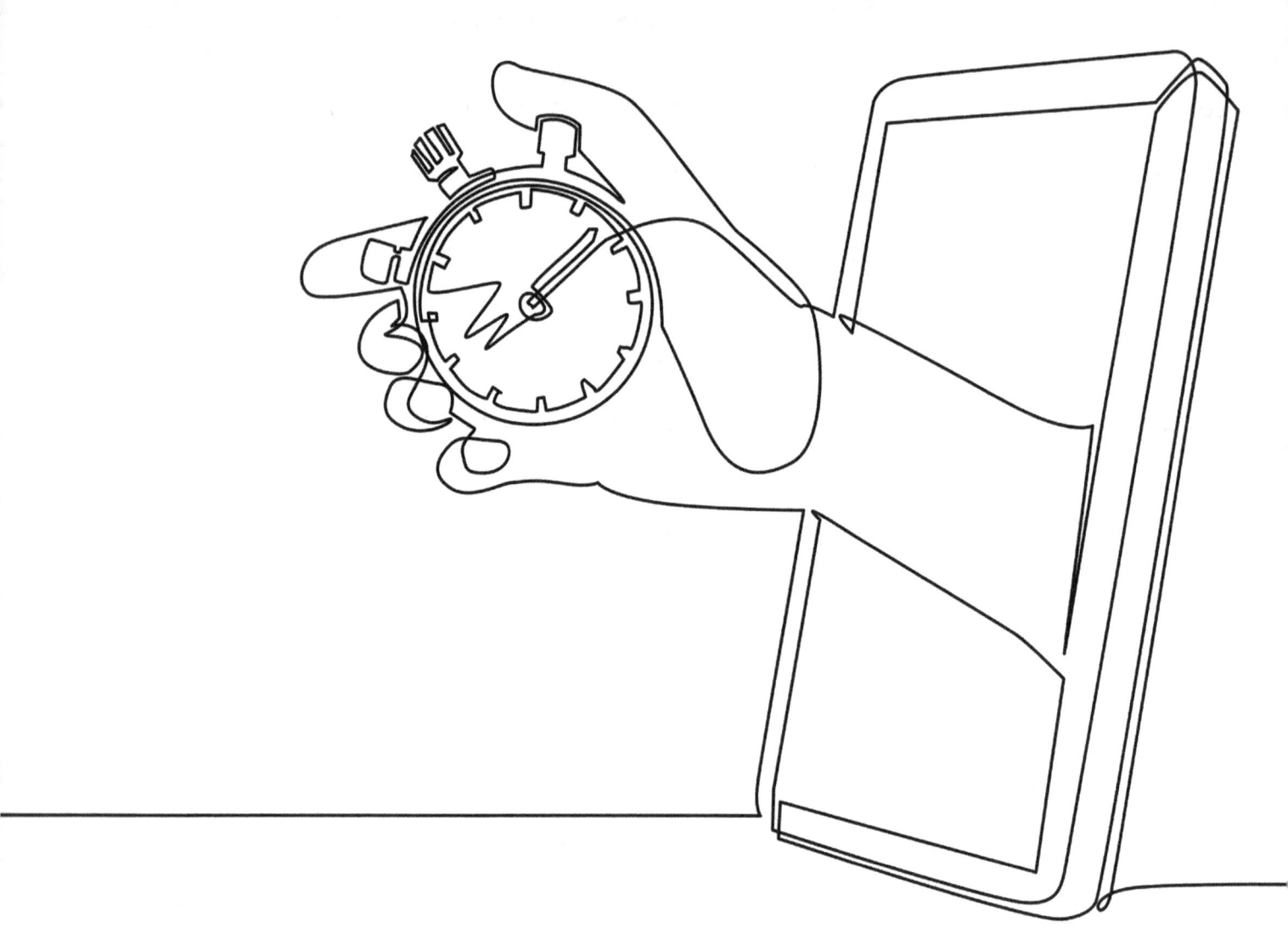

"SUCCESS IS A RESULT OF DAILY
DISCIPLINES COMPOUNDED
OVER TIME."

– DARREN HARDY

CHAPTER 5

SUBMISSION TOOLKIT

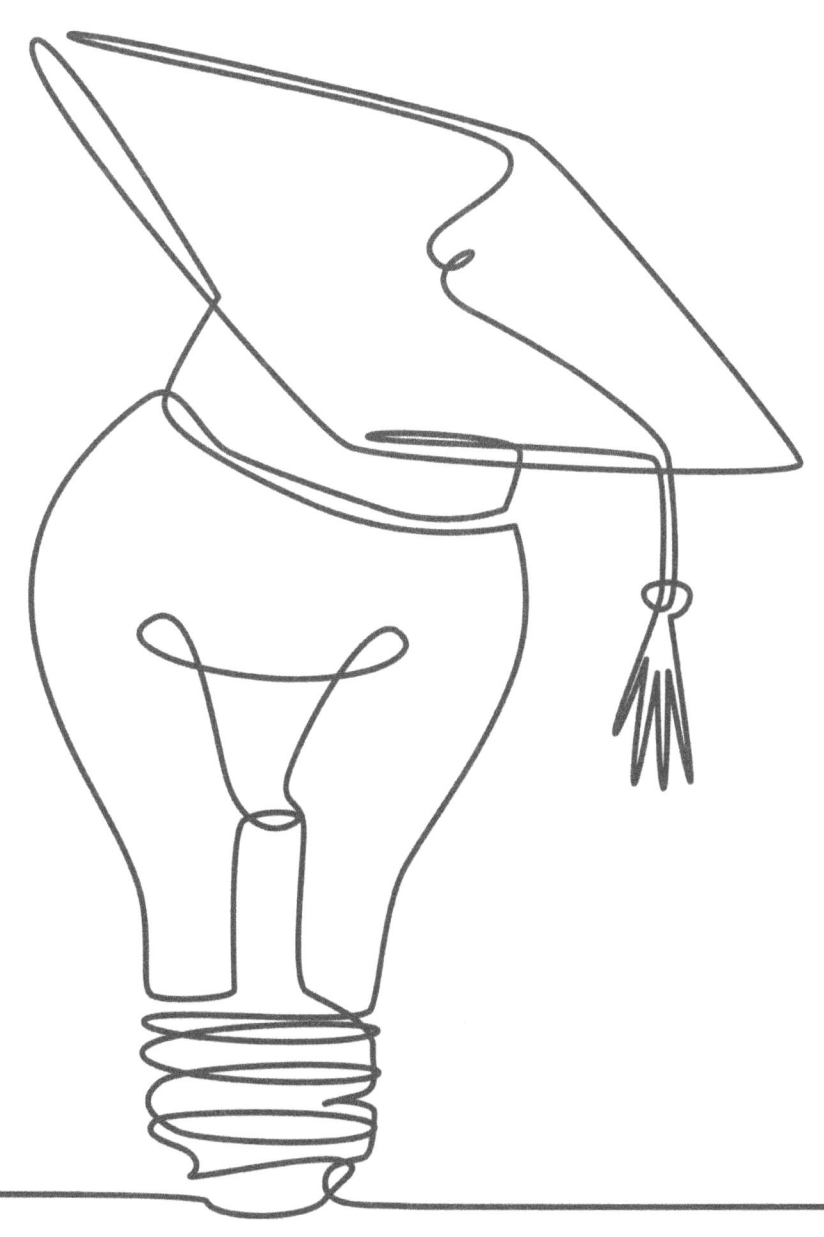

USE THIS TOOLKIT TO NAVIGATE OR ADVANCE

YOUR PROFESSIONAL CAREER.

Be prepared! Know what you need – when you need it!

PRE-NURSING AND TRANSFER CHECKLIST

UPPER DIVISION CHECKLIST

RN-TO-BSN CHECKLIST

ENTRANCE EXAMS

SCHOLARSHIP RESOURCES OR SEARCH ENGINES

GRANTS /FELLOWSHIPS

LOAN FORGIVENESS

PRE–NURSING AND TRANSFER CHECKLIST

Two Years Before Applying

STEP 1

Submit College Application

STEP 2

Start FAFSA Application

STEP 4

Take Prerequisites

STEP 3

Apply for Scholarships

STEP 5

Test Plan Prep - HESI A2, HOBET, NET, TEAS

STEP 6

Apply to Nursing School

UPPER DIVISION CHECKLIST

One Year Before Applying

STEP 1
Review Eligibility Requirements

STEP 2
Test Plan Prep - HESI A2, HOBET, NET, TEAS

STEP 4
Start Vaccination Series

STEP 3
Complete Shadow & Volunteer Opportunities

STEP 5
Be Enrolled, Accepted, or Applied to your College of Interest

STEP 6
Submit your FAFSA Initial or Renewal Application

STEP 8
Apply for Scholarships

STEP 7
Mark Important Dates

STEP 9

Gather Supplemental
Documentation

STEP 10

Apply to Nursing School

RN-TO-BSN CHECKLIST

STEP 1

Take Prerequisites

STEP 2

Submit College Application

STEP 4

Start FAFSA Application

STEP 3

Apply for Scholarships

STEP 5

If employed, inquire about Tuition Assistance and Reimbursement

STEP 6

Apply to Nursing School

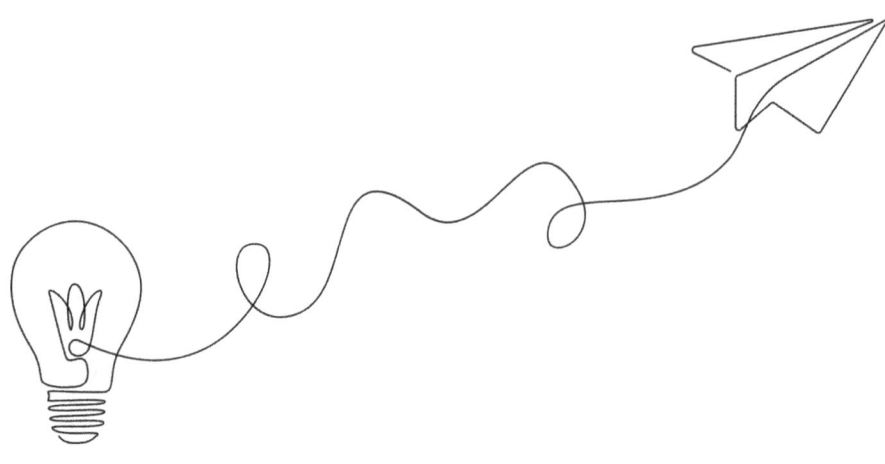

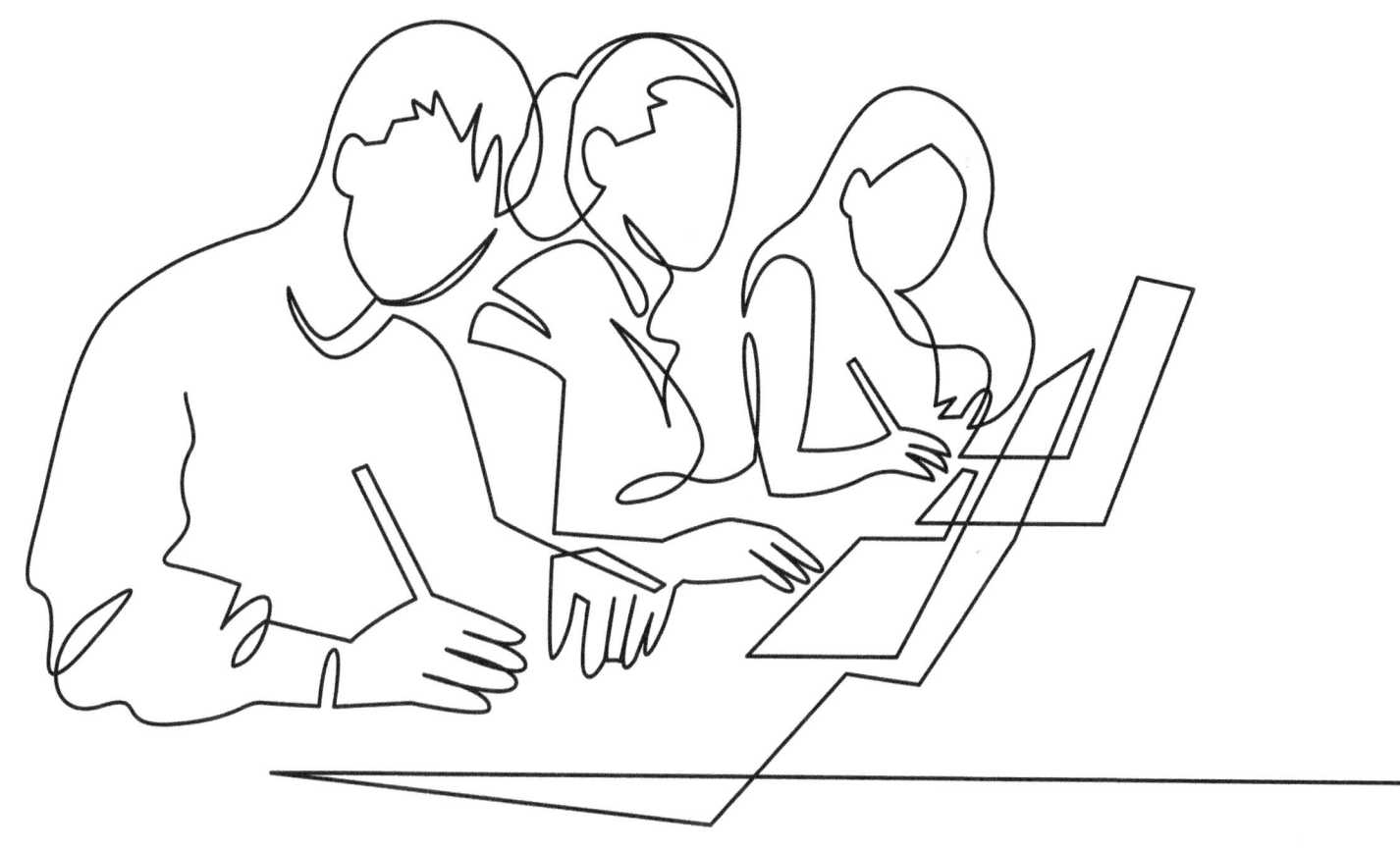

ENTRANCE EXAMS

REQUIREMENTS VARY FROM SCHOOL TO SCHOOL, BUT YOU'LL PROBABLY ENCOUNTER ONE OF THESE EXAMS FOR MOST.

HESI A2

The Health Education Systems, Inc. Exam A2 is an online exam of one to 10 sections, ranging from high school subjects to more performance-related topics, such as personality and learning styles.

HOBET

The Health Occupations Basic Entrance Test is similar to the TEAS but more comprehensive and holistic. It covers math, reading, critical thinking, test-taking skills, social interactions, stressful situations, and learning styles.

NET

The Nursing Entrance Test (NET) is another commonly used exam covering basic high school-level knowledge in reading and math. Administered through specific schools, it also aims to assess your decision-making skills, learning style, and how you handle stressful situations. Includes all NET modules (some are optional depending on your school) Reading Comprehension, Math, and English.

TEAS

The Test of Essential Academic Skills is a multiple-choice exam about subjects you learn in high school, like science, reading, English, and math. This is the test most nursing schools use, as it's a reliable indicator of a candidate's skills and knowledge.

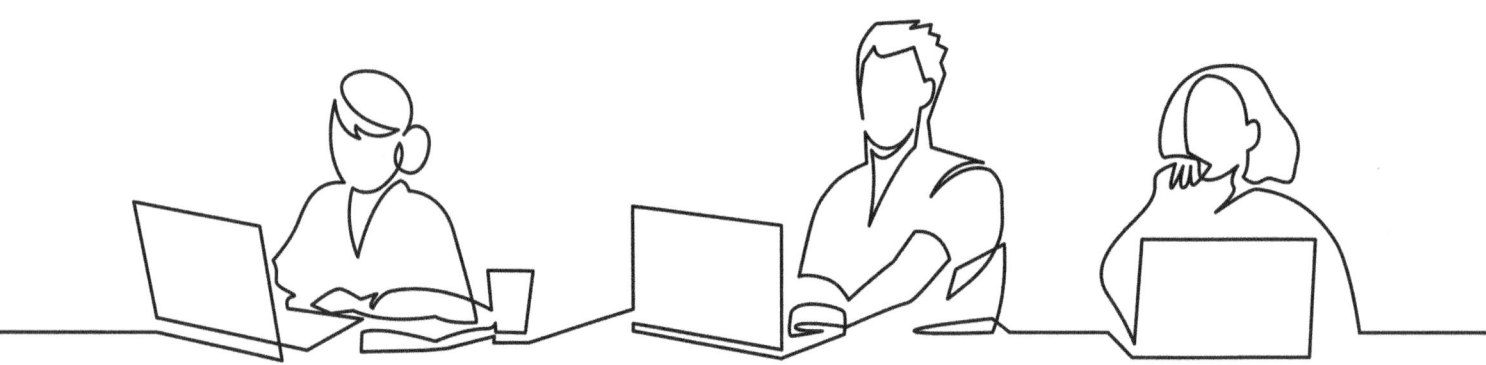

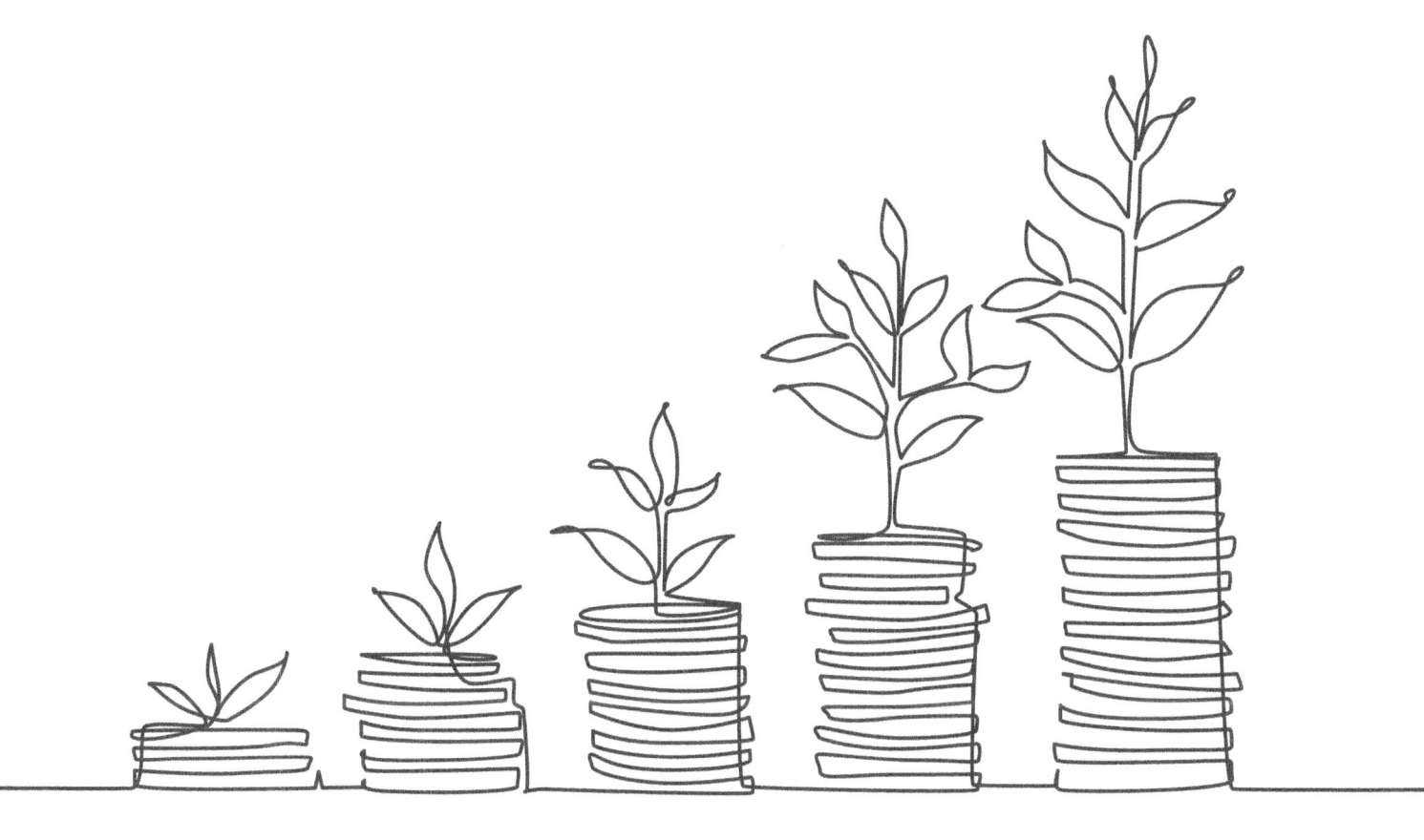

SCHOLARSHIP RESOURCES OR SEARCH ENGINES

CareerOneStop is sponsored by the US Department of Labor and has a scholarship search tool, job search function, and other helpful career resources.

Nurses' Educational Funds, Inc. distributes funds to baccalaureate-prepared registered nurses who need nursing scholarship assistance for their graduate studies.

BSN Education is a scholarship database with an emphasis on BSN-related scholarships.

Bureau of Health Professions' financial aid page offers a valuable introduction to all financial assistance programs under the Health Resources and Services Administration.

The California State Aid Commission offers a list of programs for California residents.

College Board provides an up-to-date scholarship search and advice on how to apply for a scholarship and spot a scholarship scam.

ExploreHealthCareers.org is a comprehensive Web portal that gives students a reliable and comprehensive source of accurate, up-to-date information about the health professions, including a searchable list of funding opportunities.

FastWeb is an online scholarship search.

Federal Student Aid The office of Federal Student Aid provides grants, loans, and work-study funds for college or career school. It offers more than **$150 billion** annually to help millions of students pay for higher education.

FedMoney.org is an online guide to all US federal government financial aid programs.

Campaign for action is a national nursing organization backed by the AARP Foundation, AARP, and the Robert Wood Johnson Foundation. It focuses on implementing the recommendations of the Institute of Medicine›s Future of Nursing report. The site has a list of resources available for nurses by state.

The Rural Assistance Center (RAC) is a product of the US Department of Health and Human Services› Rural Initiative, established in December 2002 as a rural health and human services information portal. RAC helps rural communities and other rural stakeholders access the full range of available programs, funding, and research that can enable them to provide quality health and human services to rural residents.

International Education Financial Aid (IEFA) scholarship search is a resource for financial aid, college scholarship, and grant information for international students wishing to study abroad.

Johnson & Johnson's Discover Nursing Web site has an extensive nursing scholarships search feature.

Maryland Higher Education Commission offers tuition reductions to Non-residents of Maryland who attend an undergraduate nursing program at a two-year or four-year Maryland public institution.

National Hartford Center of Gerontological Nursing Excellence (NHCGNE) offers the Innovation Award to a member or team of NHCGNE members and the Student Travel Awards to early career pre-doctoral and doctoral students who promote gerontological nursing excellence.

Scholarship Experts is a free and trusted scholarship resource that allows students to search for updated and accurate scholarship information.

The US Department of Education is a potential source of financial aid.

Source: Financial Aid & Scholarships (aacnnursing.org)

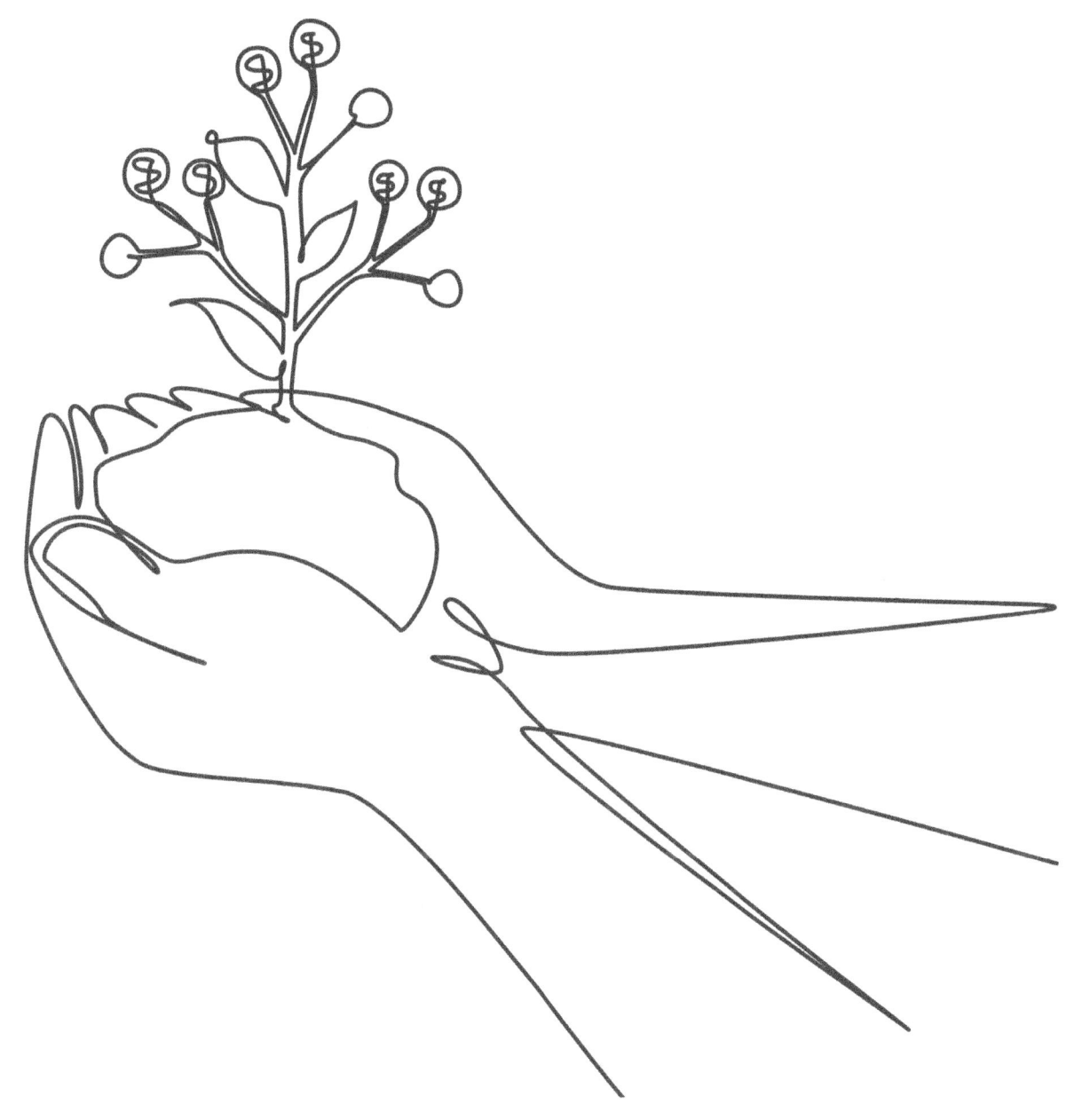

GRANTS/
FELLOWSHIPS

National Association of Neonatal Nurses (NANN) offers the Small Grants Mentee/ Mentor Program to NANN members interested in furthering their research interests or initiating their research study or evidence-based practice (EBP) project.

NCHS/Academy Health Policy Fellowship is offered to visiting scholars in health-related disciplines at the National Center for Health Statistics for 13 months to conduct studies of interest to policymakers and the health services community.

Foundation of National Student Nurses' Association, Inc. offers fellowships and grants for nursing education students.

The Oncology Nursing Society Foundation offers grants to increase the knowledge base for oncology nursing practice and prepare future oncology nurse researchers.

The Promise of Nursing Regional Faculty Fellowship offered through the Foundation of National Student Nurses› Association, Inc. awards $1,000 to $7,500 to RNs preparing for the nurse educator role to obtain their degree.

Source: Financial Aid & Scholarships (aacnnursing.org)

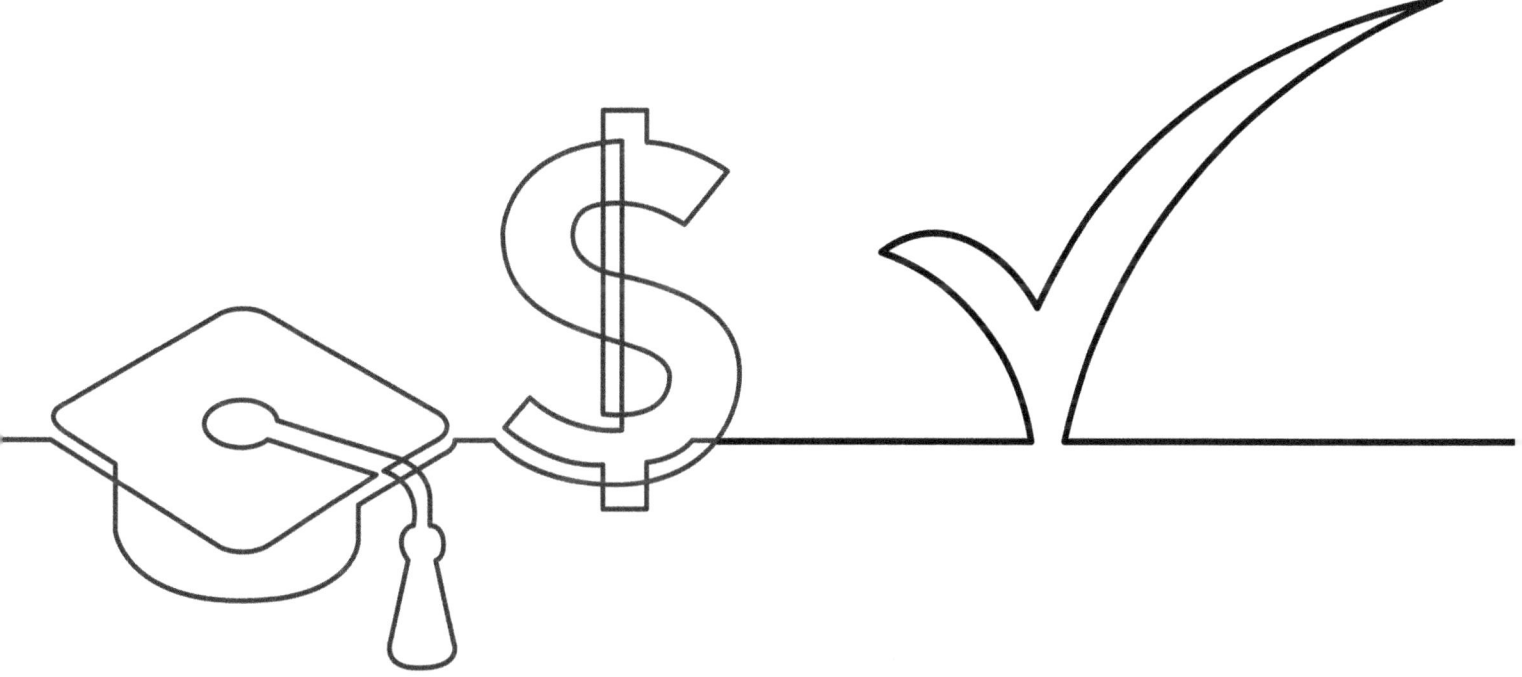

LOAN
FORGIVENESS

Army Nurse Corps Benefits provides the Health Professions Loan Repayment Program in Exchange for active-duty service in the US Army.

Disadvantaged Faculty Loan Repayment Program (FLRP) provides for repayment of education loans for individuals from disadvantaged backgrounds who agree to serve for at least two years as faculty members at eligible health professions and nursing schools.

Federal Student Aid lists loans available for college or career school.

Indian Health Service (IHS) administers a program to help repay undergraduate and graduate loans of health professionals in return for full-time clinical service in Indian health programs.

International Education Financial Aid (IEFA) offers a list of international student loans.

National Health Service Corps, a division of the US Department of Health and Human Services, offers the NHSC Loan Repayment Program for health care professionals (including Nurse Practitioners) who must work in an underserved, NHSC-approved site.

NURSE Corps Loan Repayment Program helps alleviate the shortage of nurses across the country by offering loan repayment assistance to registered nurses and advanced practice nurses, such as nurse practitioners working at Critical Shortage facilities and nurse faculty employed at accredited nursing schools. Program participants receive up to 60 percent of their qualifying student loans in exchange for a 2-year service commitment – and an additional 25 percent of their original loan balance for an optional third year.

NurseJournal.com offers financial aid resources for current and former students.

The Health Professions Education Foundation offers a list of loan repayment programs.

The Kaiser Permanente Student Financial Aid Program awards need-based nursing financial aid to students in California. Loans are available in various nursing and professional/technical specialties and may be forgiven through qualifying employment with Kaiser Permanente.

Source: Financial Aid & Scholarships (aacnnursing.org)

"EVERY TIME YOU STATE WHAT YOU WANT OR BELIEVE, YOU'RE THE FIRST TO HEAR IT. IT'S A MESSAGE TO BOTH YOU AND OTHERS ABOUT WHAT YOU THINK IS POSSIBLE. DON'T PUT A CEILING ON YOURSELF."

—OPRAH WINFREY

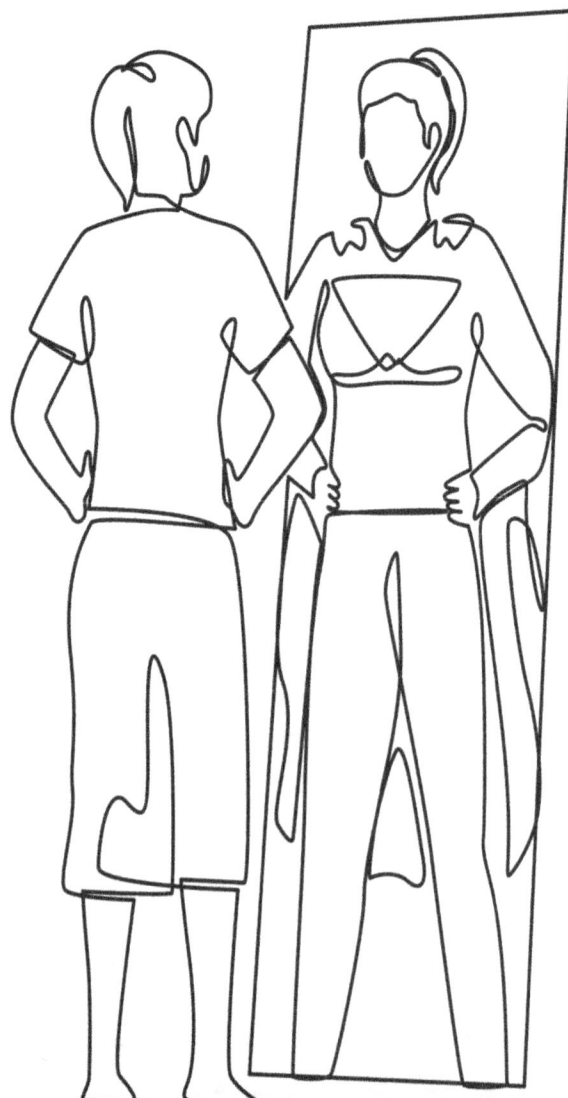

CHAPTER 6

NATIONALLY ACCREDITED NURSING PROGRAMS

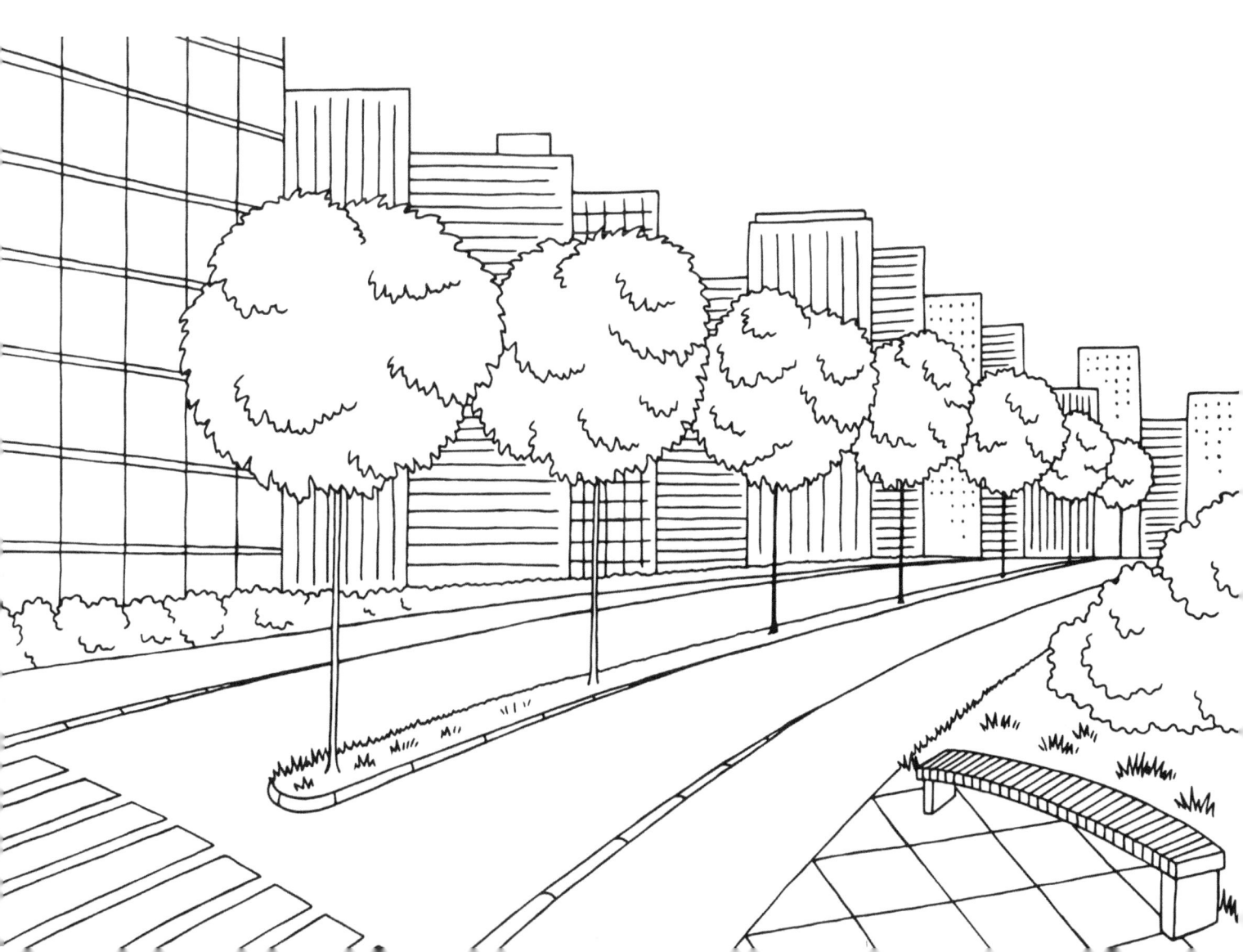

620
NURSING
PROGRAMS

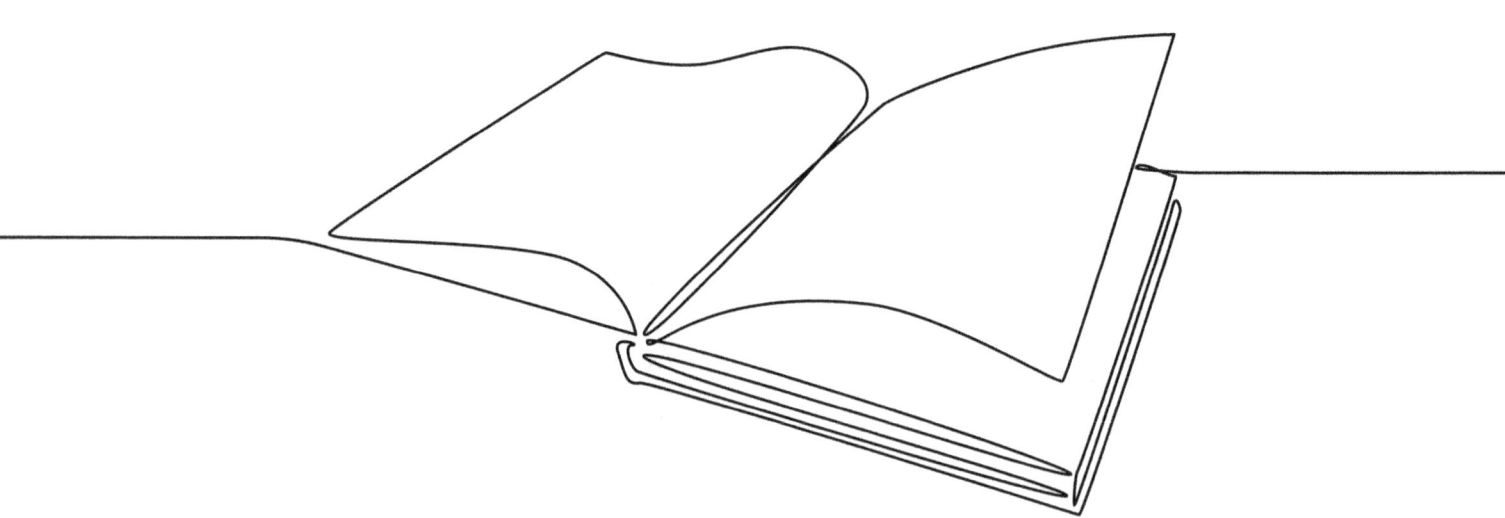

JUMPSTART YOUR QUEST

School	Location	Programs Offered
Abilene Christian University	Abilene, TX	Entry-Level BSN
Adams State University	Alamosa, CO	Entry-Level BSN RN to BSN
Adelphi University	Garden City, NY	Accelerated BSN Master's Entry-Level BSN PhD RN to BSN
AdventHealth University	Orlando, FL	Entry-Level BSN
Allen College	Waterloo, IA	Accelerated BSN Master's BSN to DNP MSN to DNP Entry-Level BSN LPN to BSN RN to BSN RN to MSN

School	Location	Programs Offered
Alvernia University	Reading, PA	Master's Entry-Level BSN LPN to BSN RN to BSN
Alverno College	Milwaukee, WI	Master's Entry-Level BSN LPN to BSN RN to BSN
American International College	Springfield, MA	Master's Entry-Level BSN RN to BSN
American University of Beirut	New York, NY	Accelerated BSN Master's Entry-Level BSN RN to BSN
American University of Health Sciences	Signal Hill, CA	Entry-Level BSN
Auburn University at Montgomery	Montgomery, AL	Master's Entry-Level BSN RN to BSN

School	Location	Programs Offered
Augusta University	Augusta, GA	BSN to DNP BSN to PhD CNL MSN to DNP Entry-Level BSN Entry-Level Master's
Augustana University	Sioux Falls, SD	CNL Entry-Level BSN
Aultman College	Canton, OH	Entry-Level BSN RN to BSN
Aurora University	Aurora, IL	Master's Entry-Level BSN RN to BSN
Averett University	Danville, VA	Entry-Level BSN
Avila University	Kansas City, MO	Entry-Level BSN
Baker College	Owosso, MI	Master's Entry-Level BSN RN to BSN

School	Location	Programs Offered
Baker University	Topeka, KS	Entry-Level BSN
Ball State University	Muncie, IN	Accelerated BSN Master's MSN to DNP Entry-Level BSN LPN to BSN RN to BSN RN to MSN
Baptist Health Sciences University	Memphis, TN	BSN to DNP Entry-Level BSN LPN to BSN RN to BSN
Barry University	Miami Shores, FL	Accelerated BSN Master's BSN to PhD MSN to DNP Entry-Level BSN PhD RN to BSN
Barton College	Wilson, NC	Entry-Level BSN RN to BSN

School	Location	Programs Offered
Baylor University	Dallas, TX	Accelerated BSN Master's BSN to DNP MSN to DNP Entry-Level BSN
Belhaven University	Jackson, MS	Entry-Level BSN RN to BSN
Bellarmine University	Louisville, KY	Accelerated BSN Master's MSN to DNP Entry-Level BSN RN to BSN
Bellin College	Green Bay, WI	Accelerated BSN Master's Entry-Level BSN RN to BSN
Belmont University	Nashville, TN	Accelerated BSN Master's BSN to DNP MSN to DNP Entry-Level BSN RN to BSN

School	Location	Programs Offered
Bemidji State University	Bemidji, MN	Entry-Level BSN RN to BSN
Benedictine College	Atchinson, KS	Entry-Level BSN
Berea College	Berea, KY	Entry-Level BSN
Berry College	Mount Berry, GA	Entry-Level BSN
Bethel College of Kansas	North Newton, KS	Entry-Level BSN
Bethel University of Minnesota	St. Paul, MN	Master's Entry-Level BSN RN to BSN
Bethel University of Tennessee	McKenzie, TN	Entry-Level BSN

School	Location	Programs Offered
Binghamton University	Binghamton, NY	Accelerated BSN BSN to DNP BSN to PhD MSN to DNP Entry-Level BSN
Biola University	La Mirada, CA	Entry-Level BSN LPN to BSN
Blessing-Rieman College of Nursing & Health Sciences	Quincy, IL	Accelerated BSN Master's Entry-Level BSN LPN to BSN RN to BSN
Bloomfield College	Bloomfield, NJ	Entry-Level BSN RN to BSN
Bloomsburg University	Bloomsburg, PA	Master's Entry-Level BSN Entry-Level Master's RN to BSN
Boise State University	Boise, ID	Master's MSN to DNP Entry-Level BSN RN to BSN

School	Location	Programs Offered
Bon Secours Memorial	Richmond, VA	Entry-Level BSN RN to BSN
Boston College	Chestnut Hill, MA	Master's BSN to PhD Entry-Level BSN Entry-Level Master's PhD RN to MSN
Bradley University	Peoria, IL	Accelerated BSN Master's Entry-Level BSN LPN to BSN RN to BSN
Brenau University	Gainesville, GA	Master's MSN to DNP Entry-Level BSN RN to BSN RN to MSN
Briar Cliff University	Sioux City, IA	Master's MSN to DNP Entry-Level BSN RN to BSN

School	Location	Programs Offered
Brigham Young University	Provo, UT	Master's Entry-Level BSN
Brookline College	Phoenix, AZ	Accelerated BSN Master's Entry-Level BSN RN to BSN
Caldwell University	Caldwell, NJ	Accelerated BSN Entry-Level BSN RN to BSN
California Baptist University	Riverside, CA	Master's Entry-Level BSN Entry-Level Master's RN to BSN
California State University-Bakersfield	Bakersfield, CA	Master's Entry-Level BSN RN to BSN
California State University-Channel Islands	Camarillo, CA	Entry-Level BSN RN to BSN
California State University-Chico	Chico, CA	Master's Entry-Level BSN LPN to BSN RN to BSN

School	Location	Programs Offered
California State University-East Bay	Hayward, CA	Entry-Level BSN LPN to BSN RN to BSN
California State University-Fresno	Fresno, CA	MSN to DNP Entry-Level BSN LPN to BSN
California State University-Fullerton	Fullerton, CA	MSN to DNP Entry-Level BSN LPN to BSN
California State University-Long Beach	Long Beach, CA	Accelerated BSN Master's Entry-Level BSN LPN to BSN Entry-Level Master's
California State University-Los Angeles	Los Angeles, CA	MSN to DNP Entry-Level BSN LPN to BSN Entry-Level Master's
California State University-Sacramento	Sacramento, CA	Master's Entry-Level BSN RN to BSN

School	Location	Programs Offered
California State University-San Bernardino	San Bernardino, CA	Master's Entry-Level BSN LPN to BSN RN to BSN
California State University-San Marcos	San Marcos, CA	Accelerated BSN Master's CNL Entry-Level BSN LPN to BSN RN to BSN
California State University-Stanislaus	Turlock, CA	Accelerated BSN Master's Entry-Level BSN LPN to BSN RN to BSN
Calvin University	Grand Rapids, MI	Entry-Level BSN
Campbell University	Buies Creek, NC	Entry-Level BSN

School	Location	Programs Offered
Capital University	Columbus, OH	Accelerated BSN Master's Entry-Level BSN RN to BSN
Carlow University	Pittsburgh, PA	Master's MSN to DNP Entry-Level BSN RN to BSN
Carroll College- Montana	Helena, MT	Entry-Level BSN
Carroll University	Waukesha, WI	Entry-Level BSN
Carson-Newman University	Jefferson City, TN	Master's Entry-Level BSN LPN to BSN RN to BSN RN to MSN
Case Western Reserve University	Cleveland, OH	BSN to PhD MSN to DNP Entry-Level BSN Entry-Level Master's

School	Location	Programs Offered
Castleton University	Castleton, VT	Entry-Level BSN RN to BSN
Cedarville University	Cedarville, OH	Master's Entry-Level BSN RN to BSN
Central Connecticut State University	New Britain, CT	Master's Entry-Level BSN RN to BSN
Central Methodist University	Fayette, MO	Master's CNL Entry-Level BSN RN to BSN
Chamberlain University - Addison	Addison, IL	Master's MSN to DNP Entry-Level BSN LPN to BSN RN to BSN
Chamberlain University - Charlotte	Charlotte, NC	Master's MSN to DNP Entry-Level BSN LPN to BSN RN to BSN

School	Location	Programs Offered
Chamberlain University - Chicago	Chicago, IL	Master's MSN to DNP Entry-Level BSN LPN to BSN RN to BSN RN to MSN
Chamberlain University - Cleveland	Cleveland, OH	Master's MSN to DNP Entry-Level BSN LPN to BSN RN to BSN
Chamberlain University - Columbus	Columbus, OH	Master's MSN to DNP Entry-Level BSN LPN to BSN RN to BSN
Chamberlain University - Houston	Houston, TX	Master's MSN to DNP Entry-Level BSN LPN to BSN RN to BSN

School	Location	Programs Offered
Chamberlain University - Irving	Irving, TX	Master's MSN to DNP Entry-Level BSN LPN to BSN RN to BSN
Chamberlain University - Irwindale	Irwindale, CA	Accelerated BSN Entry-Level BSN
Chamberlain University - Jacksonville	Jacksonville, FL	Master's MSN to DNP Entry-Level BSN LPN to BSN RN to BSN RN to MSN
Chamberlain University - Las Vegas	Las Vegas, NV	Entry-Level BSN
Chamberlain University - Miramar	Miramar, FL	Master's MSN to DNP Entry-Level BSN LPN to BSN RN to BSN
Chamberlain University - New Orleans	Jefferson, LA	Entry-Level BSN

School	Location	Programs Offered
Chamberlain University - North Brunswick	North Brunswick, NJ	Accelerated BSN Entry-Level BSN
Chamberlain University - Pearland	Pearland, TX	Accelerated BSN Master's MSN to DNP Entry-Level BSN LPN to BSN RN to BSN
Chamberlain University - Phoenix	Phoenix, AZ	Master's MSN to DNP Entry-Level BSN LPN to BSN RN to BSN
Chamberlain University - Sacramento	Rancho Cordova, CA	Accelerated BSN Entry-Level BSN
Chamberlain University - St. Louis	St. Louis, MO	Accelerated BSN Master's MSN to DNP Entry-Level BSN LPN to BSN RN to BSN RN to MSN

School	Location	Programs Offered
Chamberlain University - Tinley Park	Tinley Park, IL	Master's MSN to DNP Entry-Level BSN LPN to BSN RN to BSN
Chamberlain University - Troy	Troy, MI	Accelerated BSN Entry-Level BSN
Chamberlain University - Vienna	Vienna, VA	Master's MSN to DNP Entry-Level BSN LPN to BSN RN to BSN
Chamberlain University Headquarters	Downers Grove, IL	Master's MSN to DNP Entry-Level BSN LPN to BSN RN to BSN
Chaminade University of Honolulu	Honolulu, HI	Accelerated BSN BSN to DNP MSN to DNP Entry-Level BSN

School	Location	Programs Offered
Charles R. Drew University of Medicine and Science	Los Angeles, CA	Master's CNL MSN to DNP Entry-Level BSN Entry-Level Master's RN to BSN
Clarke University	Dubuque, IA	Master's BSN to DNP MSN to DNP Entry-Level BSN RN to BSN
Clayton State University	Morrow, GA	Master's Entry-Level BSN RN to BSN RN to MSN
Clemson University	Clemson, SC	Accelerated BSN Master's Entry-Level BSN PhD RN to BSN

School	Location	Programs Offered
Cleveland State University	Cleveland, OH	Accelerated BSN Master's CNL Entry-Level BSN PhD RN to BSN
Coe College	Cedar Rapids, IA	Entry-Level BSN
Colby-Sawyer College	New London, NH	Master's CNL Entry-Level BSN RN to BSN
College of Mount Saint Vincent	Riverdale, NY	Accelerated BSN Master's Entry-Level BSN RN to MSN
College of Saint Benedict/Saint John's University	St. Joseph, MN	Entry-Level BSN
College of the Ozarks	Point Lookout, MO	Entry-Level BSN

School	Location	Programs Offered
Colorado Christian University	Lakewood, CO	Master's Entry-Level BSN RN to BSN
Colorado Mesa University	Grand Junction, CO	Master's BSN to DNP MSN to DNP Entry-Level BSN RN to BSN
Columbia College	Columbia, MO	Entry-Level BSN RN to BSN
Columbus State University	Columbus, GA	Master's Entry-Level BSN RN to BSN
Concordia College - Minnesota	Moorhead, MN	Accelerated BSN Entry-Level BSN
Concordia University Texas	Austin, TX	Accelerated BSN Entry-Level BSN RN to BSN

School	Location	Programs Offered
Concordia University Wisconsin	Mequon, WI	Master's MSN to DNP Entry-Level BSN RN to BSN RN to MSN
Concordia University-Saint Paul	St. Paul, MN	Entry-Level BSN RN to BSN
Coppin State University	Baltimore, MD	Master's MSN to DNP Entry-Level BSN RN to BSN
Cox College	Springfield, MO	Accelerated BSN Master's CNL Entry-Level BSN LPN to BSN RN to BSN
Creighton University	Omaha, NE	Accelerated BSN Master's BSN to DNP CNL MSN to DNP Entry-Level BSN

School	Location	Programs Offered
Crown College	St. Bonifacius, MN	Entry-Level BSN RN to BSN
Cumberland University	Lebanon, TN	Master's Entry-Level BSN RN to BSN
CUNY School of Professional Studies	New York, NY	Entry-Level BSN Entry-Level Master's RN to BSN
Curry College	Milton, MA	Accelerated BSN Master's Entry-Level BSN RN to BSN
D'Youville University	Buffalo, NY	Master's MSN to DNP Entry-Level BSN RN to BSN RN to MSN
Dakota Wesleyan University	Mitchell, SD	Entry-Level BSN LPN to BSN RN to BSN
Davenport University	Grand Rapids, MI	Master's Entry-Level BSN RN to BSN

School	Location	Programs Offered
Delta State University	Cleveland, MS	Master's BSN to DNP Entry-Level BSN RN to BSN
DeSales University	Center Valley, PA	Accelerated BSN Master's MSN to DNP Entry-Level BSN RN to BSN RN to MSN
Dominican College of Blauvelt	Orangeburg, NY	Accelerated BSN Master's MSN to DNP Entry-Level BSN LPN to BSN RN to BSN
Dominican University of California	San Rafael, CA	CNL Entry-Level BSN
Dominican University of Illinois	River Forest, IL	Entry-Level BSN
Dordt University	Sioux Center, IA	Entry-Level BSN

School	Location	Programs Offered
Drexel University	Philadelphia, PA	Accelerated BSN
		Master's
		CNL
		MSN to DNP
		Entry-Level BSN
		PhD
		RN to BSN
		RN to MSN
Duquesne University	Pittsburgh, PA	Accelerated BSN
		Master's
		MSN to DNP
		Entry-Level BSN
		PhD
Eagle Gate College	Layton, UT	Master's
		Entry-Level BSN
		Entry-Level Master's
		RN to BSN
East Carolina University	Greenville, NC	Master's
		BSN to PhD
		Entry-Level BSN
		PhD
		RN to BSN

School	Location	Programs Offered
East Tennessee State University	Johnson City, TN	Accelerated BSN Master's BSN to DNP MSN to DNP Entry-Level BSN LPN to BSN PhD RN to BSN
East Texas Baptist University	Marshall, TX	Entry-Level BSN RN to BSN
Eastern Illinois University	Charleston, IL	Entry-Level BSN RN to BSN
Eastern Kentucky University	Richmond, KY	Accelerated BSN Master's MSN to DNP Entry-Level BSN RN to BSN

School	Location	Programs Offered
Eastern Mennonite University	Harrisonburg, VA	Accelerated BSN Master's MSN to DNP Entry-Level BSN LPN to BSN RN to BSN
Eastern Michigan University	Ypsilanti, MI	Accelerated BSN Master's BSN to DNP MSN to DNP Entry-Level BSN RN to BSN
Eastern University	St. Davids, PA	Accelerated BSN Entry-Level BSN RN to BSN
Edgewood College	Madison, WI	Accelerated BSN Master's BSN to DNP MSN to DNP Entry-Level BSN

School	Location	Programs Offered
Edinboro University	Edinboro, PA	Accelerated BSN Master's MSN to DNP Entry-Level BSN RN to BSN
Elmhurst University	Elmhurst, IL	Master's CNL Entry-Level BSN Entry-Level Master's RN to BSN
Elms College	Chicopee, MA	Accelerated BSN Master's BSN to DNP MSN to DNP Entry-Level BSN
Emory University	Atlanta, GA	Accelerated BSN Master's BSN to PhD Entry-Level BSN Entry-Level Master's PhD RN to MSN

School	Location	Programs Offered
Fairfield University	Fairfield, CT	Accelerated BSN Master's BSN to DNP CNL MSN to DNP Entry-Level BSN RN to BSN
Fairleigh Dickinson University	Teaneck, NJ	Accelerated BSN Master's BSN to DNP MSN to DNP Entry-Level BSN RN to BSN RN to MSN
Farmingdale State College	Farmingdale, NY	Entry-Level BSN RN to BSN
Felician University	Lodi, NJ	Accelerated BSN Master's MSN to DNP Entry-Level BSN RN to BSN

School	Location	Programs Offered
School	Location	Programs Offered
Finlandia University	Hancock, MI	Entry-Level BSN RN to BSN
Fitchburg State University	Fitchburg, MA	Master's Entry-Level BSN LPN to BSN RN to BSN
Florida Atlantic University	Boca Raton, FL	Accelerated BSN Master's BSN to DNP BSN to PhD CNL MSN to DNP Entry-Level BSN PhD RN to BSN
Florida Gulf Coast University	Fort Myers, FL	Master's BSN to DNP MSN to DNP Entry-Level BSN

School	Location	Programs Offered
Florida International University	Miami, FL	Accelerated BSN BSN to PhD MSN to DNP Entry-Level BSN PhD
Florida Southern College	Lakeland, FL	Master's MSN to DNP Entry-Level BSN
Florida State University	Tallahassee, FL	BSN to DNP MSN to DNP Entry-Level BSN
Fort Hays State University	Hays, KS	Master's Entry-Level BSN RN to BSN
Freed-Hardeman University	Henderson, TN	Entry-Level BSN RN to BSN
Fresno Pacific University	Fresno, CA	Master's Entry-Level BSN RN to BSN

School	Location	Programs Offered
Gannon University	Erie, PA	Master's MSN to DNP Entry-Level BSN RN to BSN RN to MSN
George Fox University	Newberg, OR	Entry-Level BSN
George Mason University	Fairfax, VA	Accelerated BSN BSN to DNP CNL MSN to DNP Entry-Level BSN PhD
Georgetown University	Washington, DC	Accelerated BSN Master's BSN to DNP CNL MSN to DNP Entry-Level BSN
Georgia College & State University	Milledgeville, GA	Master's MSN to DNP Entry-Level BSN RN to BSN

School	Location	Programs Offered
Georgia Southern University	Savannah, GA	MSN to DNP Entry-Level BSN LPN to BSN RN to BSN RN to MSN
Georgia Southwestern State University	Americus, GA	Accelerated BSN Master's Entry-Level BSN LPN to BSN RN to BSN
Georgia State University	Atlanta, GA	Accelerated BSN Master's BSN to PhD Entry-Level BSN PhD RN to MSN
Georgian Court University	Lakewood, NJ	Accelerated BSN Entry-Level BSN

School	Location	Programs Offered
Goldfarb School of Nursing at Barnes-Jewish College	St. Louis, MO	Accelerated BSN Master's MSN to DNP Entry-Level BSN PhD RN to BSN
Gonzaga University	Spokane, WA	Master's MSN to DNP Entry-Level BSN RN to MSN
Goshen College	Goshen, IN	Master's Entry-Level BSN RN to BSN
Graceland University	Independence, MO	Master's MSN to DNP Entry-Level BSN RN to BSN RN to MSN
Grand Canyon University	Phoenix, AZ	Accelerated BSN Master's Entry-Level BSN RN to BSN

School	Location	Programs Offered
Grand Valley State University	Grand Rapids, MI	Accelerated BSN
		Master's
		BSN to DNP
		CNL
		MSN to DNP
		Entry-Level BSN
		RN to BSN
Grand View University	Des Moines, IA	Master's
		CNL
		Entry-Level BSN
		LPN to BSN
		RN to BSN
Gustavus Adolphus College	Saint Peter, MN	Entry-Level BSN
Hampton University	Hampton, VA	Master's
		Entry-Level BSN
		LPN to BSN
		PhD
		RN to BSN
		RN to MSN

School	Location	Programs Offered
Harding University	Searcy, AR	Master's Entry-Level BSN LPN to BSN RN to BSN RN to MSN
Hartwick College	Oneonta, NY	Accelerated BSN Entry-Level BSN LPN to BSN RN to BSN
Hawaii Pacific University	Honolulu, HI	Master's Entry-Level BSN LPN to BSN RN to BSN RN to MSN
Henderson State University	Arkadelphia, AR	Entry-Level BSN
Heritage University	Toppenish, WA	Entry-Level BSN
Herzing University Akron	Akron, OH	Entry-Level BSN RN to BSN

School	Location	Programs Offered
Herzing University Atlanta	Atlanta, GA	Master's Entry-Level BSN RN to BSN
Herzing University Brookfield	Brookfield, WI	Master's Entry-Level BSN RN to BSN
Herzing University Kenosha	Kenosha, WI	Master's Entry-Level BSN RN to BSN
Herzing University Minneapolis	St. Louis Park, MN	Master's Entry-Level BSN RN to BSN
Herzing University Orlando	Winter Park, FL	Master's Entry-Level BSN LPN to BSN RN to BSN
Hiram College	Hiram, OH	Entry-Level BSN

School	Location	Programs Offered
Holy Family University	Philadelphia, PA	Accelerated BSN Master's BSN to DNP MSN to DNP Entry-Level BSN RN to BSN
Hood College	Frederick, MD	Entry-Level BSN RN to BSN
Hope College	Holland, MI	Entry-Level BSN
Howard University	Washington, DC	Master's Entry-Level BSN LPN to BSN RN to BSN
Huntington University	Huntington, IN	Entry-Level BSN RN to BSN
Husson University	Bangor, ME	Master's Entry-Level BSN RN to BSN

School	Location	Programs Offered
Idaho State University	Pocatello, ID	Accelerated BSN Master's CNL Entry-Level BSN LPN to BSN RN to BSN RN to MSN
Illinois State University	Normal, IL	Accelerated BSN Master's CNL Entry-Level BSN PhD RN to BSN
Illinois Wesleyan University	Bloomington, IL	Entry-Level BSN
Immaculata University	Immaculata, PA	Master's Entry-Level BSN RN to BSN
Indiana University Fort Wayne	Fort Wayne, IN	Master's Entry-Level BSN LPN to BSN RN to BSN

School	Location	Programs Offered
Indiana University Kokomo	Kokomo, IN	Master's Entry-Level BSN RN to BSN
Indiana University of Pennsylvania	Indiana, PA	Master's Entry-Level BSN LPN to BSN PhD
Indiana University South Bend	South Bend, IN	Accelerated BSN Master's Entry-Level BSN RN to BSN
Indiana University Southeast	New Albany, IN	Entry-Level BSN RN to BSN
Indiana University-Purdue University (Columbus)	Columbus, IN	Accelerated BSN Entry-Level BSN RN to BSN
Indiana University-Purdue University (Indianapolis)	Indianapolis, IN	Accelerated BSN BSN to PhD MSN to DNP Entry-Level BSN PhD

School	Location	Programs Offered
Indiana Wesleyan University	Marion, IN	Accelerated BSN Master's MSN to DNP Entry-Level BSN RN to BSN
Jacksonville State University	Jacksonville, AL	Master's Entry-Level BSN RN to BSN
Jacksonville University	Jacksonville, FL	Accelerated BSN Master's MSN to DNP Entry-Level BSN RN to BSN
James Madison University	Harrisonburg, VA	Master's CNL MSN to DNP Entry-Level BSN RN to BSN RN to MSN
John Brown University	Siloam Springs, AR	Entry-Level BSN

School	Location	Programs Offered
Johns Hopkins University	Baltimore, MD	Accelerated BSN BSN to PhD MSN to DNP Entry-Level BSN
Joyce University	Draper, UT	Master's Entry-Level BSN RN to BSN
Kansas Wesleyan University	Salina, KS	Entry-Level BSN RN to BSN
Keene State College	Keene, NH	Entry-Level BSN RN to BSN
Keiser University	Ft. Lauderdale, FL	Accelerated BSN Master's MSN to DNP Entry-Level BSN RN to BSN
Kennesaw State University	Kennesaw, GA	Accelerated BSN Master's Entry-Level BSN PhD RN to BSN

School	Location	Programs Offered
Kent State University	Kent, OH	Accelerated BSN Master's BSN to PhD MSN to DNP Entry-Level BSN LPN to BSN PhD RN to BSN
Kentucky Christian University	Grayson, KY	Master's Entry-Level BSN RN to BSN
King University	Bristol, TN	Master's Entry-Level BSN RN to BSN
La Salle University	Philadelphia, PA	Master's CNL MSN to DNP Entry-Level BSN RN to BSN
Lakeview College of Nursing	Danville, IL	Accelerated BSN Entry-Level BSN LPN to BSN RN to BSN

School	Location	Programs Offered
Lander University	Greenwood, SC	Master's CNL Entry-Level BSN RN to BSN
Lawrence Technological University	Southfield, MI	Entry-Level BSN
Lebanese American University	New York, NY	Entry-Level BSN RN to BSN
Lee University	Cleveland, TN	Entry-Level BSN
Lees-McRae College	Banner Elk, NC	Entry-Level BSN
Lehman College	Bronx, NY	Accelerated BSN Entry-Level BSN RN to BSN
Lenoir-Rhyne University	Hickory, NC	Master's Entry-Level BSN RN to BSN
LeTourneau University	Longview, TX	Entry-Level BSN

School	Location	Programs Offered
Lewis University	Romeoville, IL	Accelerated BSN Master's MSN to DNP Entry-Level BSN RN to BSN
Lewis-Clark State College	Lewiston, ID	Entry-Level BSN LPN to BSN RN to BSN
Liberty University	Lynchburg, VA	Master's Entry-Level BSN LPN to BSN RN to BSN
Lincoln University - Pennsylvania	Lincoln University, PA	Entry-Level BSN RN to BSN
Lindsey Wilson College	Columbia, KY	Entry-Level BSN
Linfield University	Portland, OR	Accelerated BSN Entry-Level BSN RN to BSN

School	Location	Programs Offered
Loma Linda University	Loma Linda, CA	Accelerated BSN MSN to DNP Entry-Level BSN LPN to BSN PhD
Long Island University - LIU Brooklyn	Brooklyn, NY	Accelerated BSN Master's Entry-Level BSN RN to BSN RN to MSN
Longwood University	Farmville, VA	Entry-Level BSN
Louisiana College	Pineville, LA	Accelerated BSN Entry-Level BSN
Louisiana State University Health Sciences Ctr	New Orleans, LA	Accelerated BSN MSN to DNP Entry-Level BSN LPN to BSN PhD

School	Location	Programs Offered
Lourdes University	Sylvania, OH	Entry-Level BSN LPN to BSN RN to BSN RN to MSN
Loyola University Chicago	Maywood, IL	Accelerated BSN BSN to DNP BSN to PhD MSN to DNP Entry-Level BSN
Luther College	Decorah, IA	Entry-Level BSN
Madonna University	Livonia, MI	Master's MSN to DNP Entry-Level BSN LPN to BSN RN to BSN RN to MSN
Malone University	Canton, OH	Master's Entry-Level BSN RN to BSN
Maranatha Baptist University	Watertown, WI	Entry-Level BSN

School	Location	Programs Offered
Marian University	Fond du Lac, WI	Master's Entry-Level BSN RN to BSN
Marian University- Indiana	Indianapolis, IN	Accelerated BSN Entry-Level BSN RN to BSN
Marquette University	Milwaukee, WI	BSN to DNP BSN to PhD CNL MSN to DNP Entry-Level BSN Entry-Level Master's
Mars Hill University	Mars Hill, NC	Entry-Level BSN RN to BSN
Marymount University	Arlington, VA	Accelerated BSN Master's BSN to DNP MSN to DNP Entry-Level BSN RN to BSN

School	Location	Programs Offered
Maryville University-Saint Louis	St. Louis, MO	Master's MSN to DNP Entry-Level BSN RN to BSN
Marywood University	Scranton, PA	Master's Entry-Level BSN LPN to BSN
McNeese State University	Lake Charles, LA	Master's Entry-Level BSN LPN to BSN RN to BSN
MCPHS University	Boston, MA	Accelerated BSN Master's Entry-Level BSN RN to BSN RN to MSN
Mercer University	Atlanta, GA	Master's MSN to DNP Entry-Level BSN PhD RN to BSN

School	Location	Programs Offered
Mercy College	Dobbs Ferry, NY	Master's Entry-Level BSN RN to BSN RN to MSN
Mercy College of Ohio	Toledo, OH	Entry-Level BSN RN to BSN
Messiah University	Mechanicsburg, PA	Master's BSN to DNP MSN to DNP Entry-Level BSN RN to MSN
Methodist College	Peoria, IL	Accelerated BSN Master's Entry-Level BSN RN to BSN
Methodist University	Fayetteville, NC	Entry-Level BSN
Miami University	Hamilton, OH	Entry-Level BSN RN to BSN

School	Location	Programs Offered
Michigan State University	East Lansing, MI	Accelerated BSN Master's BSN to PhD Entry-Level BSN PhD RN to BSN
MidAmerica Nazarene University	Olathe, KS	Accelerated BSN Master's Entry-Level BSN RN to BSN RN to MSN
Middle Tennessee State University	Murfreesboro, TN	Master's Entry-Level BSN LPN to BSN RN to BSN RN to MSN
Midwestern State University	Wichita Falls, TX	Master's Entry-Level BSN RN to BSN RN to MSN
Milligan University	Milligan, TN	Entry-Level BSN RN to BSN

School	Location	Programs Offered
Millikin University	Decatur, IL	Master's BSN to DNP CNL MSN to DNP Entry-Level BSN Entry-Level Master's RN to BSN
Milwaukee School of Engineering	Milwaukee, WI	Accelerated BSN Master's Entry-Level BSN
Minnesota State University Mankato	Mankato, MN	Master's BSN to DNP MSN to DNP Entry-Level BSN RN to BSN
Misericordia University	Dallas, PA	Accelerated BSN Master's BSN to DNP MSN to DNP Entry-Level BSN RN to BSN
Mississippi College	Clinton, MS	Entry-Level BSN RN to BSN

School	Location	Programs Offered
Mississippi University for Women	Columbus, MS	Master's Entry-Level BSN RN to BSN
Missouri State University	Springfield, MO	Master's MSN to DNP Entry-Level BSN LPN to BSN RN to BSN
Missouri Western State University	St. Joseph, MO	Master's Entry-Level BSN RN to BSN
Molloy College	Rockville Centre, NY	Accelerated BSN Master's Entry-Level BSN LPN to BSN PhD RN to BSN
Monmouth University	West Long Branch, NJ	Master's MSN to DNP Entry-Level BSN RN to BSN RN to MSN

School	Location	Programs Offered
Montana State University-Bozeman	Bozeman, MT	Accelerated BSN Master's BSN to DNP CNL MSN to DNP Entry-Level BSN LPN to BSN
Moravian University	Bethlehem, PA	Master's CNL Entry-Level BSN RN to BSN
Morehead State University	Morehead, KY	Master's Entry-Level BSN RN to BSN
Morgan State University	Baltimore, MD	Master's Entry-Level BSN PhD
Morningside University	Sioux City, IA	Entry-Level BSN LPN to BSN

School	Location	Programs Offered
Mount Carmel College of Nursing	Columbus, OH	Accelerated BSN Master's MSN to DNP Entry-Level BSN RN to BSN
Mount Marty University	Yankton, SD	Master's MSN to DNP Entry-Level BSN LPN to BSN RN to BSN
Mount Mercy University	Cedar Rapids, IA	Master's Entry-Level BSN RN to BSN
Mount Saint Joseph University	Cincinnati, OH	Master's CNL MSN to DNP Entry-Level BSN LPN to BSN Entry-Level Master's RN to BSN

School	Location	Programs Offered
Mount Saint Mary College- New York	Newburgh, NY	Master's MSN to DNP Entry-Level BSN LPN to BSN RN to BSN
Mount Saint Mary's University	Los Angeles, CA	Accelerated BSN Master's Entry-Level BSN LPN to BSN RN to BSN RN to MSN
Mount Vernon Nazarene University	Mount Vernon, OH	Entry-Level BSN
Murray State University	Murray, KY	Master's BSN to DNP MSN to DNP Entry-Level BSN RN to BSN
Muskingum University	New Concord, OH	Entry-Level BSN RN to BSN

School	Location	Programs Offered
National University	San Diego, CA	Accelerated BSN Master's MSN to DNP Entry-Level BSN LPN to BSN RN to BSN
Nazareth College	Rochester, NY	Entry-Level BSN LPN to BSN RN to BSN
Nebraska Methodist College	Omaha, NE	Accelerated BSN Master's Entry-Level BSN LPN to BSN RN to BSN RN to MSN
Nebraska Wesleyan University	Lincoln, NE	Master's Entry-Level BSN RN to BSN
Nevada State College	Henderson, NV	Accelerated BSN Entry-Level BSN RN to BSN

School	Location	Programs Offered
New Mexico State University	Las Cruces, NM	Master's BSN to DNP MSN to DNP Entry-Level BSN PhD RN to BSN
New York Institute of Technology	Old Westbury, NY	Entry-Level BSN
New York University	New York, NY	Accelerated BSN Master's MSN to DNP Entry-Level BSN PhD
Niagara University	Niagara, NY	Accelerated BSN Entry-Level BSN RN to BSN
Nicholls State University	Thibodaux, LA	Master's Entry-Level BSN LPN to BSN RN to BSN

School	Location	Programs Offered
Nightingale College	Salt Lake City, UT	Accelerated BSN Master's Entry-Level BSN RN to BSN
North Dakota State University	Fargo, ND	Master's BSN to DNP MSN to DNP Entry-Level BSN LPN to BSN RN to BSN
North Park University	Chicago, IL	Master's Entry-Level BSN RN to BSN
Northeastern University	Boston, MA	Accelerated BSN BSN to PhD MSN to DNP Entry-Level BSN Entry-Level Master's
Northern Arizona University	Flagstaff, AZ	Accelerated BSN Master's MSN to DNP Entry-Level BSN RN to BSN

School	Location	Programs Offered
Northern Illinois University	DeKalb, IL	Master's MSN to DNP Entry-Level BSN RN to BSN
Northern Kentucky University	Highland Heights, KY	Accelerated BSN Master's MSN to DNP Entry-Level BSN RN to BSN
Northern Michigan University	Marquette, MI	Master's Entry-Level BSN LPN to BSN RN to BSN
Northwest Nazarene University	Nampa, ID	Master's Entry-Level BSN RN to MSN
Northwest University	Kirkland, WA	Entry-Level BSN
Northwestern College	Orange City, IA	Entry-Level BSN

School	Location	Programs Offered
Northwestern Oklahoma State University	Alva, OK	BSN to DNP Entry-Level BSN LPN to BSN RN to BSN
Northwestern State University	Shreveport, LA	Master's BSN to DNP MSN to DNP Entry-Level BSN LPN to BSN RN to BSN
Norwich University	Northfield, VT	Master's Entry-Level BSN
Notre Dame of Maryland University	Baltimore, MD	Master's Entry-Level BSN RN to BSN RN to MSN
Nova Southeastern University	Ft Lauderdale, FL	Master's MSN to DNP Entry-Level BSN PhD RN to BSN RN to MSN

School	Location	Programs Offered
Nyack College	New York, NY	Entry-Level BSN
Oak Point University	Chicago, IL	Accelerated BSN Master's CNL Entry-Level BSN RN to BSN RN to MSN
Oakland University	Rochester, MI	Accelerated BSN Master's BSN to DNP CNL MSN to DNP Entry-Level BSN RN to BSN
Ohio Northern University	Ada, OH	Entry-Level BSN RN to BSN
Ohio University	Athens, OH	Accelerated BSN Master's Entry-Level BSN LPN to BSN RN to BSN

School	Location	Programs Offered
Oklahoma Baptist University	Shawnee, OK	Master's Entry-Level BSN LPN to BSN RN to BSN
Oklahoma Christian University	Oklahoma City, OK	Entry-Level BSN
Oklahoma Wesleyan University	Bartlesville, OK	Entry-Level BSN LPN to BSN RN to BSN
Old Dominion University	Virginia Beach, VA	Accelerated BSN Master's MSN to DNP Entry-Level BSN RN to BSN
Olivet Nazarene University	Bourbonnais, IL	Master's Entry-Level BSN RN to BSN
Oral Roberts University	Tulsa, OK	Master's MSN to DNP Entry-Level BSN RN to BSN

School	Location	Programs Offered
Oregon Health and Science University	Portland, OR	Accelerated BSN BSN to DNP MSN to DNP Entry-Level BSN PhD
Otterbein University	Westerville, OH	Master's CNL MSN to DNP Entry-Level BSN RN to MSN
Pace University	Pleasantville, NY	Accelerated BSN Master's CNL MSN to DNP Entry-Level BSN RN to BSN
Pacific Lutheran University	Tacoma, WA	CNL Entry-Level BSN LPN to BSN Entry-Level Master's RN to BSN

School	Location	Programs Offered
Palm Beach Atlantic University	West Palm Beach, FL	Master's BSN to DNP MSN to DNP Entry-Level BSN
Park University	Parkville, MO	Entry-Level BSN RN to BSN
Patty Hanks Shelton School of Nursing	Abilene, TX	Accelerated BSN Master's Entry-Level BSN RN to BSN
Pennsylvania State University	University Park, PA	Accelerated BSN Master's BSN to PhD Entry-Level BSN PhD RN to BSN
Pfeiffer University	Misenheimer, NC	Entry-Level BSN RN to BSN

School	Location	Programs Offered
Pittsburg State University	Pittsburg, KS	Master's BSN to DNP MSN to DNP Entry-Level BSN RN to BSN
Plymouth State University	Plymouth, NH	Entry-Level BSN RN to BSN
Point Loma Nazarene University	San Diego, CA	Master's Entry-Level BSN LPN to BSN RN to BSN RN to MSN
Prairie View A & M University	Houston, TX	Master's MSN to DNP Entry-Level BSN LPN to BSN RN to BSN
Presentation College	Aberdeen, SD	Master's Entry-Level BSN LPN to BSN RN to BSN

School	Location	Programs Offered
Provo College	Provo, UT	Entry-Level BSN RN to BSN
Purdue University	West Lafayette, IN	Accelerated BSN Entry-Level BSN
Queens University of Charlotte	Charlotte, NC	Accelerated BSN Master's CNL Entry-Level BSN RN to BSN RN to MSN
Quinnipiac University	Hamden, CT	Accelerated BSN Master's BSN to DNP MSN to DNP Entry-Level BSN
Radford University	Radford, VA	Master's BSN to DNP MSN to DNP Entry-Level BSN RN to BSN

School	Location	Programs Offered
Rasmussen University	Bloomington, MN	Accelerated BSN Master's Entry-Level BSN RN to BSN
Regis University	Denver, CO	Accelerated BSN Master's MSN to DNP Entry-Level BSN RN to BSN RN to MSN
Research College of Nursing	Kansas City, MO	Accelerated BSN Master's CNL Entry-Level BSN RN to MSN
Rhode Island College	Providence, RI	Master's Entry-Level BSN RN to BSN
Robert Morris University	Moon Township, PA	Accelerated BSN BSN to DNP MSN to DNP Entry-Level BSN RN to MSN

School	Location	Programs Offered
Roberts Wesleyan College	Rochester, NY	Master's Entry-Level BSN RN to BSN
Rochester University	Rochester Hills, MI	Entry-Level BSN RN to BSN
Rockhurst University	Kansas City, MO	Master's Entry-Level BSN RN to BSN
Russell Sage College	Troy, NY	Accelerated BSN Master's Entry-Level BSN PhD RN to BSN
Rutgers University - Camden	Camden, NJ	Accelerated BSN MSN to DNP Entry-Level BSN RN to BSN
Sacred Heart University	Fairfield, CT	Master's CNL MSN to DNP Entry-Level BSN RN to BSN RN to MSN

School	Location	Programs Offered
Saginaw Valley State University	University Center, MI	BSN to DNP CNL MSN to DNP Entry-Level BSN RN to BSN
Saint Ambrose University	Davenport, IA	Entry-Level BSN RN to BSN
Saint Anselm College	Manchester, NH	Entry-Level BSN RN to BSN
Saint Anthony College of Nursing	Rockford, IL	Master's CNL Entry-Level BSN RN to BSN
Saint Cloud State University	St. Cloud, MN	Entry-Level BSN
Saint Francis College	Brooklyn, NY	Entry-Level BSN RN to BSN

School	Location	Programs Offered
Saint Francis Medical Center College of Nursing	Peoria, IL	Master's CNL MSN to DNP Entry-Level BSN RN to BSN
Saint Francis University	Loretto, PA	Master's Entry-Level BSN
Saint John Fisher College	Rochester, NY	Master's MSN to DNP Entry-Level BSN RN to BSN RN to MSN
Saint Joseph's College of Maine	Standish, ME	Master's Entry-Level BSN RN to BSN
Saint Louis University	Saint Louis, MO	Accelerated BSN BSN to DNP CNL MSN to DNP Entry-Level BSN Entry-Level Master's

School	Location	Programs Offered
Saint Mary's College- Indiana	Notre Dame, IN	Accelerated BSN BSN to DNP Entry-Level BSN
Saint Olaf College	Northfield, MN	Entry-Level BSN
Saint Peter's University	Jersey City, NJ	Master's MSN to DNP Entry-Level BSN RN to BSN
Saint Thomas University	Miami Gardens, FL	Entry-Level BSN RN to BSN RN to MSN
Saint Xavier University	Chicago, IL	Master's CNL Entry-Level BSN LPN to BSN
Salem State University	Salem, MA	Master's Entry-Level BSN LPN to BSN RN to BSN RN to MSN

School	Location	Programs Offered
Salisbury University	Salisbury, MD	Accelerated BSN Master's MSN to DNP Entry-Level BSN RN to BSN RN to MSN
Salve Regina University	Newport, RI	Accelerated BSN Entry-Level BSN RN to BSN
Sam Houston State University	The Woodlands, TX	Entry-Level BSN LPN to BSN RN to BSN
Samford University	Birmingham, AL	Accelerated BSN Master's MSN to DNP Entry-Level BSN RN to MSN
Samuel Merritt University	Oakland, CA	Accelerated BSN Master's MSN to DNP Entry-Level BSN Entry-Level Master's

School	Location	Programs Offered
San Diego State University	San Diego, CA	Accelerated BSN Master's Entry-Level BSN RN to BSN
San Francisco State University	San Francisco, CA	Master's Entry-Level BSN Entry-Level Master's
San Jose State University	San Jose, CA	Master's MSN to DNP Entry-Level BSN RN to BSN
Schreiner University	Kerrville, TX	Entry-Level BSN
Seattle Pacific University	Seattle, WA	CNL MSN to DNP Entry-Level BSN
Seattle University	Seattle, WA	Master's MSN to DNP Entry-Level BSN Entry-Level Master's

School	Location	Programs Offered
Sentara College of Health Sciences	Chesapeake, VA	Master's Entry-Level BSN LPN to BSN RN to BSN
Seton Hall University	Nutley, NJ	Accelerated BSN BSN to DNP CNL MSN to DNP Entry-Level BSN Entry-Level Master's
Shenandoah University	Winchester, VA	Accelerated BSN Master's BSN to DNP MSN to DNP Entry-Level BSN RN to MSN
Shepherd University	Shepherdstown, WV	BSN to DNP Entry-Level BSN RN to BSN
Shorter University	Rome, GA	Entry-Level BSN

School	Location	Programs Offered
Siena Heights University	Adrian, MI	Entry-Level BSN RN to BSN
Simmons University	Boston, MA	Accelerated BSN MSN to DNP Entry-Level BSN LPN to BSN Entry-Level Master's
South Dakota State University	Brookings, SD	Accelerated BSN BSN to DNP CNL MSN to DNP Entry-Level BSN PhD
South University	Savannah, GA	Master's Entry-Level BSN RN to BSN RN to MSN
Southeast Missouri State University	Cape Girardeau, MO	Accelerated BSN Master's Entry-Level BSN RN to BSN

School	Location	Programs Offered
Southeastern Louisiana University	Hammond, LA	Accelerated BSN Master's MSN to DNP Entry-Level BSN LPN to BSN RN to BSN
Southeastern University	Lakeland, FL	Entry-Level BSN RN to BSN
Stony Brook University	Stony Brook, NY	Accelerated BSN MSN to DNP Entry-Level BSN RN to BSN RN to MSN
Stratford University	Alexandria, VA	Entry-Level BSN RN to BSN
SUNY Brockport	Brockport, NY	Entry-Level BSN RN to BSN
SUNY Plattsburgh	Plattsburgh, NY	Entry-Level BSN RN to BSN

School	Location	Programs Offered
Tarleton State University	Stephenville, TX	Master's Entry-Level BSN LPN to BSN RN to BSN RN to MSN
Temple University	Philadelphia, PA	Master's BSN to DNP CNL MSN to DNP Entry-Level BSN RN to BSN
Tennessee Technological University	Cookeville, TN	Accelerated BSN Master's CNL Entry-Level BSN RN to BSN
Tennessee Wesleyan University	Knoxville, TN	Entry-Level BSN RN to BSN
Texas A&M University Health Science Center	Bryan, TX	Accelerated BSN Master's Entry-Level BSN RN to BSN

School	Location	Programs Offered
Texas A&M University-Commerce	Commerce, TX	Master's Entry-Level BSN RN to BSN
Texas A&M University-Corpus Christi	Corpus Christi, TX	Accelerated BSN Master's MSN to DNP Entry-Level BSN RN to BSN RN to MSN
Texas A&M University-Texarkana	Texarkana, TX	Master's Entry-Level BSN RN to BSN
Texas Christian University	Fort Worth, TX	Accelerated BSN Master's BSN to DNP CNL MSN to DNP Entry-Level BSN RN to MSN
Texas Lutheran University	Sequin, TX	Entry-Level BSN

School	Location	Programs Offered
Texas State University	Round Rock, TX	Master's Entry-Level BSN
Texas Tech University Health Sciences Center	Lubbock, TX	Accelerated BSN BSN to DNP MSN to DNP Entry-Level BSN RN to BSN RN to MSN
Texas Tech University Health Sciences Center-El Paso	El Paso, TX	Accelerated BSN Entry-Level BSN
Texas Woman's University	Denton, TX	Master's CNL MSN to DNP Entry-Level BSN PhD RN to BSN RN to MSN
The Catholic University of America	Washington, DC	Accelerated BSN Master's MSN to DNP Entry-Level BSN PhD

School	Location	Programs Offered
The Christ College of Nursing and Health Sciences	Cincinnati, OH	Accelerated BSN Entry-Level BSN RN to BSN
The College of New Jersey	Ewing, NJ	Master's CNL Entry-Level BSN RN to BSN RN to MSN
The College of Saint Scholastica	Duluth, MN	Accelerated BSN BSN to DNP MSN to DNP Entry-Level BSN RN to BSN
The Ohio State University	Columbus, OH	BSN to PhD CNL MSN to DNP Entry-Level BSN Entry-Level Master's
The University of Akron	Akron, OH	Accelerated BSN BSN to PhD MSN to DNP Entry-Level BSN LPN to BSN

School	Location	Programs Offered
The University of Alabama	Tuscaloosa, AL	Master's CNL MSN to DNP Entry-Level BSN RN to BSN RN to MSN
The University of Alabama in Huntsville	Huntsville, AL	Master's MSN to DNP Entry-Level BSN PhD RN to BSN
The University of Findlay	Findlay, OH	Entry-Level BSN
The University of South Dakota	Sioux Falls, SD	Entry-Level BSN RN to BSN
The University of Tampa	Tampa, FL	Master's Entry-Level BSN RN to BSN

School	Location	Programs Offered
Thomas Jefferson University	Philadelphia, PA	Accelerated BSN Master's MSN to DNP Entry-Level BSN RN to BSN
Toccoa Falls College	Toccoa Falls, GA	Entry-Level BSN
Touro University	Henderson, NV	Accelerated BSN Master's MSN to DNP Entry-Level BSN RN to BSN
Towson University	Towson, MD	Master's Entry-Level BSN RN to BSN
Trinity Christian College	Palos Heights, IL	Entry-Level BSN
Trinity College of Nursing and Health Sciences	Rock Island, IL	Accelerated BSN Master's Entry-Level BSN LPN to BSN RN to BSN

School	Location	Programs Offered
Trinity Washington University	Washington, DC	Accelerated BSN Master's Entry-Level BSN RN to BSN
Truman State University	Kirksville, MO	Accelerated BSN Entry-Level BSN
Tusculum University	Greeneville, TN	Accelerated BSN Master's Entry-Level BSN RN to BSN
Union College-Kentucky	Barbourville, KY	Entry-Level BSN RN to BSN
Union College-Nebraska	Lincoln, NE	Entry-Level BSN LPN to BSN
Union University-Tennessee	Jackson, TN	Accelerated BSN MSN to DNP Entry-Level BSN LPN to BSN RN to BSN
Universidad Central de Bayamon	Bayamon, PR	Entry-Level BSN

School	Location	Programs Offered
Universidad de Puerto Rico	San Juan, PR	Master's Entry-Level BSN PhD
University at Buffalo-SUNY	Buffalo, NY	Accelerated BSN Master's BSN to DNP BSN to PhD MSN to DNP Entry-Level BSN PhD RN to BSN
University of Alabama at Birmingham	Birmingham, AL	BSN to PhD CNL MSN to DNP Entry-Level BSN Entry-Level Master's
University of Alaska Anchorage	Anchorage, AK	Master's Entry-Level BSN RN to BSN
University of Arizona	Tucson, AZ	BSN to DNP BSN to PhD MSN to DNP Entry-Level BSN Entry-Level Master's

School	Location	Programs Offered
University of Arkansas at Pine Bluff	Pine Bluff, AR	Entry-Level BSN LPN to BSN RN to BSN
University of Arkansas for Medical Sciences	Little Rock, AR	Master's BSN to PhD Entry-Level BSN LPN to BSN PhD RN to BSN RN to MSN
University of Arkansas- Fort Smith	Fort Smith, AR	Entry-Level BSN RN to BSN
University of Arkansas-Fayetteville	Fayetteville, AR	Master's Entry-Level BSN LPN to BSN RN to BSN
University of California-Irvine	Irvine, CA	Master's BSN to DNP MSN to DNP Entry-Level BSN

School	Location	Programs Offered
University of California-Los Angeles	Los Angeles, CA	Master's BSN to PhD CNL Entry-Level BSN Entry-Level Master's PhD
University of Central Arkansas	Conway, AR	Master's CNL Entry-Level BSN LPN to BSN RN to BSN RN to MSN
University of Central Florida	Orlando, FL	Accelerated BSN BSN to DNP CNL MSN to DNP Entry-Level BSN PhD
University of Central Missouri	Warrensburg, MO	Master's Entry-Level BSN RN to BSN
University of Central Oklahoma	Edmond, OK	Entry-Level BSN LPN to BSN RN to BSN

School	Location	Programs Offered
University of Cincinnati	Cincinnati, OH	Master's BSN to DNP BSN to PhD MSN to DNP Entry-Level BSN Entry-Level Master's PhD RN to BSN
University of Colorado--Anschutz	Aurora, CO	Accelerated BSN BSN to PhD MSN to DNP Entry-Level BSN PhD
University of Colorado--Colorado Springs	Colorado Springs, CO	Accelerated BSN Master's MSN to DNP Entry-Level BSN RN to BSN
University of Delaware	Newark, DE	Accelerated BSN Master's Entry-Level BSN PhD RN to BSN RN to MSN

School	Location	Programs Offered
University of Detroit Mercy	Detroit, MI	Accelerated BSN Master's CNL MSN to DNP Entry-Level BSN RN to BSN
University of Dubuque	Dubuque, IA	Entry-Level BSN
University of Hawaii at Hilo	Hilo, HI	BSN to DNP MSN to DNP Entry-Level BSN RN to BSN
University of Hawaii at Manoa	Honolulu, HI	Master's Entry-Level BSN Entry-Level Master's PhD
University of Indianapolis	Indianapolis, IN	Master's Entry-Level BSN RN to BSN

School	Location	Programs Offered
University of Iowa	Iowa City, IA	BSN to DNP BSN to PhD CNL MSN to DNP Entry-Level BSN
University of Kansas	Kansas City, KS	Master's BSN to DNP BSN to PhD CNL MSN to DNP Entry-Level BSN PhD RN to BSN RN to MSN
University of Kentucky	Lexington, KY	Accelerated BSN BSN to DNP BSN to PhD MSN to DNP Entry-Level BSN
University of Louisiana at Lafayette	Lafayette, LA	Master's MSN to DNP Entry-Level BSN RN to BSN

School	Location	Programs Offered
University of Louisiana at Monroe	Monroe, LA	Master's CNL Entry-Level BSN LPN to BSN RN to BSN
University of Louisville	Louisville, KY	Accelerated BSN Master's BSN to PhD Entry-Level BSN Entry-Level Master's PhD RN to BSN
University of Lynchburg	Lynchburg, VA	Master's CNL Entry-Level BSN RN to MSN
University of Maine	Orono, ME	Master's Entry-Level BSN RN to BSN RN to MSN
University of Maine-Fort Kent	Fort Kent, ME	Accelerated BSN Entry-Level BSN RN to BSN

School	Location	Programs Offered
University of Mary	Bismarck, ND	Master's Entry-Level BSN LPN to BSN RN to BSN RN to MSN
University of Mary Hardin-Baylor	Belton, TX	Master's Entry-Level BSN RN to BSN
University of Maryland	Baltimore, MD	BSN to PhD CNL MSN to DNP Entry-Level BSN Entry-Level Master's RN to BSN
University of Massachusetts-Boston	Boston, MA	Accelerated BSN BSN to PhD MSN to DNP Entry-Level BSN PhD
University of Massachusetts-Dartmouth	North Dartmouth, MA	BSN to DNP MSN to DNP Entry-Level BSN PhD RN to BSN

School	Location	Programs Offered
University of Massachusetts-Lowell	Lowell, MA	Master's MSN to DNP Entry-Level BSN PhD
University of Memphis	Memphis, TN	Accelerated BSN Master's Entry-Level BSN RN to BSN
University of Miami	Coral Gables, FL	Accelerated BSN BSN to PhD MSN to DNP Entry-Level BSN PhD
University of Michigan	Ann Arbor, MI	Accelerated BSN BSN to PhD MSN to DNP Entry-Level BSN PhD
University of Michigan-Flint	Flint, MI	Accelerated BSN BSN to DNP MSN to DNP Entry-Level BSN RN to BSN

School	Location	Programs Offered
University of Minnesota	Minneapolis, MN	BSN to DNP BSN to PhD CNL MSN to DNP Entry-Level BSN
University of Mississippi Medical Center	Jackson, MS	Accelerated BSN Master's MSN to DNP Entry-Level BSN PhD RN to BSN RN to MSN
University of Missouri-Columbia	Columbia, MO	Accelerated BSN Master's BSN to DNP BSN to PhD MSN to DNP Entry-Level BSN PhD RN to BSN

School	Location	Programs Offered
University of Missouri-Kansas City	Kansas City, MO	Accelerated BSN BSN to PhD MSN to DNP Entry-Level BSN PhD
University of Missouri-St. Louis	St. Louis, MO	Accelerated BSN BSN to PhD MSN to DNP Entry-Level BSN PhD
University of Mobile	Mobile, AL	Accelerated BSN Master's Entry-Level BSN RN to BSN
University of Mount Union	Alliance, OH	Entry-Level BSN
University of Nebraska Medical Center	Omaha, NE	Accelerated BSN BSN to PhD MSN to DNP Entry-Level BSN PhD RN to BSN

School	Location	Programs Offered
University of Nevada-Las Vegas	Las Vegas, NV	Master's MSN to DNP Entry-Level BSN PhD
University of Nevada-Reno	Reno, NV	Master's CNL MSN to DNP Entry-Level BSN RN to BSN
University of New Hampshire	Durham, NH	Master's CNL MSN to DNP Entry-Level BSN Entry-Level Master's
University of New Mexico	Albuquerque, NM	Accelerated BSN Master's BSN to PhD Entry-Level BSN PhD RN to BSN

School	Location	Programs Offered
University of North Alabama	Florence, AL	Accelerated BSN Master's Entry-Level BSN RN to BSN RN to MSN
University of North Carolina-Chapel Hill	Chapel Hill, NC	Accelerated BSN BSN to PhD CNL Entry-Level BSN PhD RN to BSN
University of North Carolina-Charlotte	Charlotte, NC	Master's Entry-Level BSN RN to BSN RN to MSN
University of North Carolina-Greensboro	Greensboro, NC	Master's Entry-Level BSN PhD RN to BSN
University of North Carolina-Pembroke	Pembroke, NC	Master's CNL Entry-Level BSN RN to BSN

School	Location	Programs Offered
University of North Carolina-Wilmington	Wilmington, NC	Master's Entry-Level BSN RN to BSN
University of North Dakota	Grand Forks, ND	Accelerated BSN Master's Entry-Level BSN LPN to BSN PhD RN to BSN
University of North Florida	Jacksonville, FL	Accelerated BSN CNL MSN to DNP Entry-Level BSN RN to BSN RN to MSN
University of Northern Colorado	Greeley, CO	Accelerated BSN Master's BSN to DNP CNL MSN to DNP Entry-Level BSN PhD RN to BSN

School	Location	Programs Offered
University of Northwestern-Saint Paul	Saint Paul, MN	Accelerated BSN Entry-Level BSN
University of Oklahoma	Oklahoma City, OK	Accelerated BSN BSN to PhD CNL MSN to DNP Entry-Level BSN
University of Pennsylvania	Philadelphia, PA	Accelerated BSN Master's BSN to PhD Entry-Level BSN PhD RN to BSN
University of Pittsburgh	Pittsburgh, PA	Accelerated BSN BSN to DNP BSN to PhD CNL MSN to DNP Entry-Level BSN

School	Location	Programs Offered
University of Portland	Portland, OR	Master's BSN to DNP CNL MSN to DNP Entry-Level BSN
University of Rhode Island	Kingston, RI	Master's CNL MSN to DNP Entry-Level BSN PhD RN to BSN
University of Saint Francis-Indiana	Fort Wayne, IN	Master's Entry-Level BSN RN to BSN RN to MSN
University of Saint Francis-Illinois	Joliet, IL	Master's MSN to DNP Entry-Level BSN RN to BSN
University of Saint Joseph	West Hartford, CT	Accelerated BSN Master's MSN to DNP Entry-Level BSN RN to BSN

School	Location	Programs Offered
University of Saint Mary	Leavenworth, KS	Accelerated BSN Master's Entry-Level BSN RN to BSN
University of Saint Thomas	Houston, TX	Entry-Level BSN
University of San Francisco	San Francisco, CA	BSN to DNP CNL MSN to DNP Entry-Level BSN Entry-Level Master's
University of Scranton	Scranton, PA	Master's Entry-Level BSN LPN to BSN RN to BSN RN to MSN
University of Sioux Falls	Sioux Falls, SD	Accelerated BSN Entry-Level BSN RN to BSN

School	Location	Programs Offered
University of South Alabama	Mobile, AL	Accelerated BSN
		BSN to DNP
		CNL
		MSN to DNP
		Entry-Level BSN
		Entry-Level Master's
University of South Carolina	Columbia, SC	Master's
		BSN to DNP
		BSN to PhD
		MSN to DNP
		Entry-Level BSN
		PhD
University of South Carolina Aiken	Aiken, SC	Entry-Level BSN
		RN to BSN
University of South Carolina Beaufort	Bluffton, SC	Entry-Level BSN
		RN to BSN
University of South Carolina Upstate	Spartanburg, SC	CNL
		Entry-Level BSN
		RN to BSN

School	Location	Programs Offered
University of South Florida	Tampa, FL	Accelerated BSN Master's BSN to DNP BSN to PhD MSN to DNP Entry-Level BSN PhD RN to BSN RN to MSN
University of Southern Indiana	Evansville, IN	Master's MSN to DNP Entry-Level BSN RN to BSN RN to MSN
University of Southern Maine	Portland, ME	Accelerated BSN CNL MSN to DNP Entry-Level BSN Entry-Level Master's

School	Location	Programs Offered
University of Southern Mississippi	Hattiesburg, MS	Master's MSN to DNP Entry-Level BSN PhD RN to BSN RN to MSN
University of Tennessee- Health Science Center	Memphis, TN	Accelerated BSN BSN to DNP BSN to PhD MSN to DNP Entry-Level BSN Entry-Level Master's RN to BSN
University of Tennessee-Chattanooga	Chattanooga, TN	Master's BSN to DNP MSN to DNP Entry-Level BSN RN to BSN
University of Tennessee-Knoxville	Knoxville, TN	Accelerated BSN BSN to PhD MSN to DNP Entry-Level BSN

School	Location	Programs Offered
University of Tennessee-Southern	Pulaski, TN	Entry-Level BSN RN to BSN
University of Texas Health Science Center-Houston	Houston, TX	Accelerated BSN Master's MSN to DNP Entry-Level BSN PhD RN to BSN
University of Texas Health Science Center-San Anto	San Antonio, TX	Accelerated BSN BSN to PhD CNL MSN to DNP Entry-Level BSN PhD
University of Texas Medical Branch	Galveston, TX	Accelerated BSN BSN to PhD CNL MSN to DNP Entry-Level BSN PhD
University of Texas Permian Basin	Odessa, TX	Entry-Level BSN RN to BSN

School	Location	Programs Offered
University of Texas Rio Grande Valley	Edinburg, TX	Master's Entry-Level BSN
University of Texas-Arlington	Arlington, TX	Accelerated BSN BSN to PhD MSN to DNP Entry-Level BSN PhD
University of Texas-Austin	Austin, TX	BSN to PhD Entry-Level BSN Entry-Level Master's PhD RN to BSN
University of Texas-El Paso	El Paso, TX	Accelerated BSN MSN to DNP Entry-Level BSN RN to BSN RN to MSN
University of Texas-Tyler	Tyler, TX	Accelerated BSN BSN to PhD Entry-Level BSN LPN to BSN PhD

School	Location	Programs Offered
University of the Incarnate Word	San Antonio, TX	Master's BSN to DNP MSN to DNP Entry-Level BSN RN to MSN
University of Toledo	Toledo, OH	Master's BSN to DNP CNL MSN to DNP Entry-Level BSN Entry-Level Master's RN to BSN
University of Utah	Salt Lake City, UT	Accelerated BSN BSN to PhD MSN to DNP Entry-Level BSN
University of Vermont	Burlington, VT	Master's BSN to DNP CNL MSN to DNP Entry-Level BSN Entry-Level Master's RN to BSN

School	Location	Programs Offered
University of Virginia	Charlottesville, VA	BSN to PhD CNL MSN to DNP Entry-Level BSN Entry-Level Master's
University of Virginia's College at Wise	Wise, VA	Entry-Level BSN RN to BSN
University of Washington	Seattle, WA	Accelerated BSN Master's BSN to DNP BSN to PhD CNL MSN to DNP Entry-Level BSN PhD RN to BSN
University of West Florida	Pensacola, FL	Master's Entry-Level BSN RN to BSN

School	Location	Programs Offered
University of West Georgia	Carrollton, GA	Master's CNL Entry-Level BSN PhD RN to BSN
University of Wisconsin-Eau Claire	Eau Claire, WI	Accelerated BSN BSN to DNP MSN to DNP Entry-Level BSN RN to BSN
University of Wisconsin-Madison	Madison, WI	Accelerated BSN BSN to DNP BSN to PhD MSN to DNP Entry-Level BSN PhD
University of Wisconsin-Milwaukee	Milwaukee, WI	BSN to DNP BSN to PhD CNL MSN to DNP Entry-Level BSN

School	Location	Programs Offered
University of Wisconsin-Oshkosh	Oshkosh, WI	Accelerated BSN BSN to DNP CNL MSN to DNP Entry-Level BSN
University of Wyoming	Laramie, WY	Accelerated BSN Master's BSN to DNP MSN to DNP Entry-Level BSN RN to BSN
Ursuline College	Pepper Pike, OH	Accelerated BSN Master's BSN to DNP MSN to DNP Entry-Level BSN RN to BSN RN to MSN
Utica University	Utica, NY	Accelerated BSN Entry-Level BSN RN to BSN

School	Location	Programs Offered
Valdosta State University	Valdosta, GA	Accelerated BSN Master's BSN to DNP MSN to DNP Entry-Level BSN
Valparaiso University	Valparaiso, IN	Accelerated BSN Master's BSN to DNP MSN to DNP Entry-Level BSN RN to BSN RN to MSN
Villanova University	Villanova, PA	Accelerated BSN Master's BSN to PhD MSN to DNP Entry-Level BSN PhD

School	Location	Programs Offered
Virginia Commonwealth University	Richmond, VA	Accelerated BSN Master's BSN to PhD CNL MSN to DNP Entry-Level BSN PhD RN to BSN
Viterbo University	LaCrosse, WI	BSN to DNP MSN to DNP Entry-Level BSN RN to BSN
Walsh University	North Canton, OH	Accelerated BSN Master's CNL MSN to DNP Entry-Level BSN RN to BSN
Warner Pacific University	Portland, OR	Entry-Level BSN

School	Location	Programs Offered
Washburn University	Topeka, KS	Master's CNL MSN to DNP Entry-Level BSN LPN to BSN RN to BSN
Washington Adventist University	Takoma Park, MD	Master's Entry-Level BSN RN to BSN
Washington State University	Spokane, WA	Master's MSN to DNP Entry-Level BSN PhD RN to BSN
Wayne State University	Detroit, MI	Accelerated BSN BSN to DNP BSN to PhD MSN to DNP Entry-Level BSN

School	Location	Programs Offered
Waynesburg University	Waynesburg, PA	Accelerated BSN Master's MSN to DNP Entry-Level BSN LPN to BSN RN to BSN
Wesleyan College-Georgia	Macon, GA	Entry-Level BSN
West Chester University	Exton, PA	Accelerated BSN Master's MSN to DNP Entry-Level BSN RN to BSN
West Coast University	Irvine, CA	Master's Entry-Level BSN LPN to BSN RN to BSN RN to MSN
West Liberty University	West Liberty, WV	Entry-Level BSN RN to BSN

School	Location	Programs Offered
West Texas A&M University	Canyon, TX	Master's Entry-Level BSN LPN to BSN RN to BSN RN to MSN
West Virginia University	Morgantown, WV	Accelerated BSN MSN to DNP Entry-Level BSN PhD RN to BSN
West Virginia Wesleyan College	Buckhannon, WV	Master's Entry-Level BSN
Western Carolina University	Cullowhee, NC	Accelerated BSN Master's BSN to DNP MSN to DNP Entry-Level BSN RN to BSN
Western Connecticut State University	Danbury, CT	Master's Entry-Level BSN RN to BSN

School	Location	Programs Offered
Western Governors University	Salt Lake City, UT	Accelerated BSN Master's CNL Entry-Level BSN RN to BSN RN to MSN
Western Illinois University	Macomb, IL	Entry-Level BSN RN to BSN
Western Kentucky University	Bowling Green, KY	Master's MSN to DNP Entry-Level BSN RN to BSN
Western Michigan University	Kalamazoo, MI	Master's Entry-Level BSN RN to BSN
Westfield State University	Westfield, MA	Entry-Level BSN RN to BSN
Westminster College--Utah	Salt Lake City, UT	Master's Entry-Level BSN

School	Location	Programs Offered
Wheeling University	Wheeling, WV	Accelerated BSN Master's Entry-Level BSN RN to BSN RN to MSN
Wichita State University	Wichita, KS	Accelerated BSN Master's BSN to DNP MSN to DNP Entry-Level BSN LPN to BSN RN to BSN RN to MSN
Widener University	Chester, PA	Master's BSN to PhD MSN to DNP Entry-Level BSN PhD RN to BSN

School	Location	Programs Offered
Wilkes University	Wilkes-Barre, PA	Accelerated BSN
		Master's
		BSN to DNP
		MSN to DNP
		Entry-Level BSN
		LPN to BSN
		RN to BSN
		RN to MSN
William Carey University--Hattiesburg	Hattiesburg, MS	Master's
		Entry-Level BSN
		PhD
		RN to BSN
William Jewell College	Liberty, MO	Accelerated BSN
		Entry-Level BSN
William Paterson University	Wayne, NJ	Accelerated BSN
		Master's
		MSN to DNP
		Entry-Level BSN
		RN to BSN

School	Location	Programs Offered
Winona State University	Winona, MN	Master's MSN to DNP Entry-Level BSN RN to BSN RN to MSN
Winston-Salem State University	Winston-Salem, NC	Accelerated BSN Master's Entry-Level BSN LPN to BSN RN to BSN
Wisconsin Lutheran College	Milwaukee, WI	Entry-Level BSN
Worcester State University	Worcester, MA	Master's Entry-Level BSN LPN to BSN RN to BSN RN to MSN
Wright State University	Dayton, OH	Accelerated BSN Master's CNL MSN to DNP Entry-Level BSN RN to BSN

School	Location	Programs Offered
Xavier University	Cincinnati, OH	Master's CNL Entry-Level BSN Entry-Level Master's RN to MSN
York College of Pennsylvania	York, PA	Master's MSN to DNP Entry-Level BSN LPN to BSN RN to BSN RN to MSN
Youngstown State University	Youngstown, OH	Master's Entry-Level BSN RN to BSN

SCHOOLS:

TASKS TO DO:

NOTES:

SCHOOLS:

TASKS TO DO:

NOTES:

"BE PASSIONATE AND MOVE FORWARD WITH GUSTO. EVERY SINGLE HOUR OF EVERY SINGLE DAY UNTIL YOU REACH YOUR GOAL."

–AVA DUVERNAY

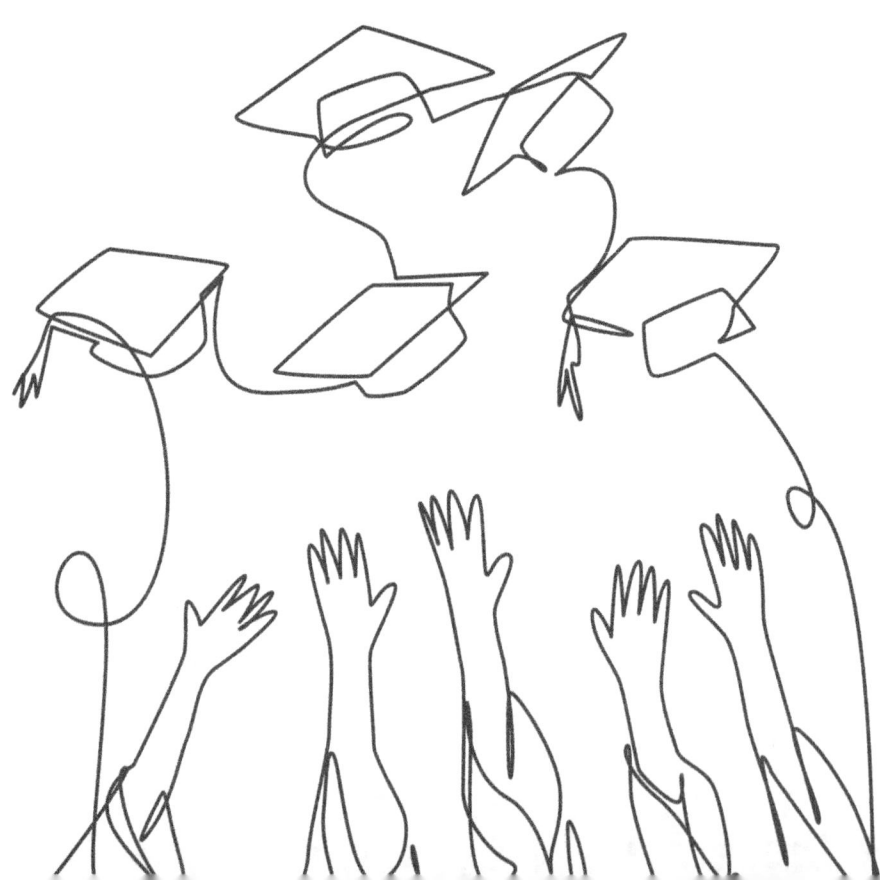

CHAPTER 7
FINAL WORDS

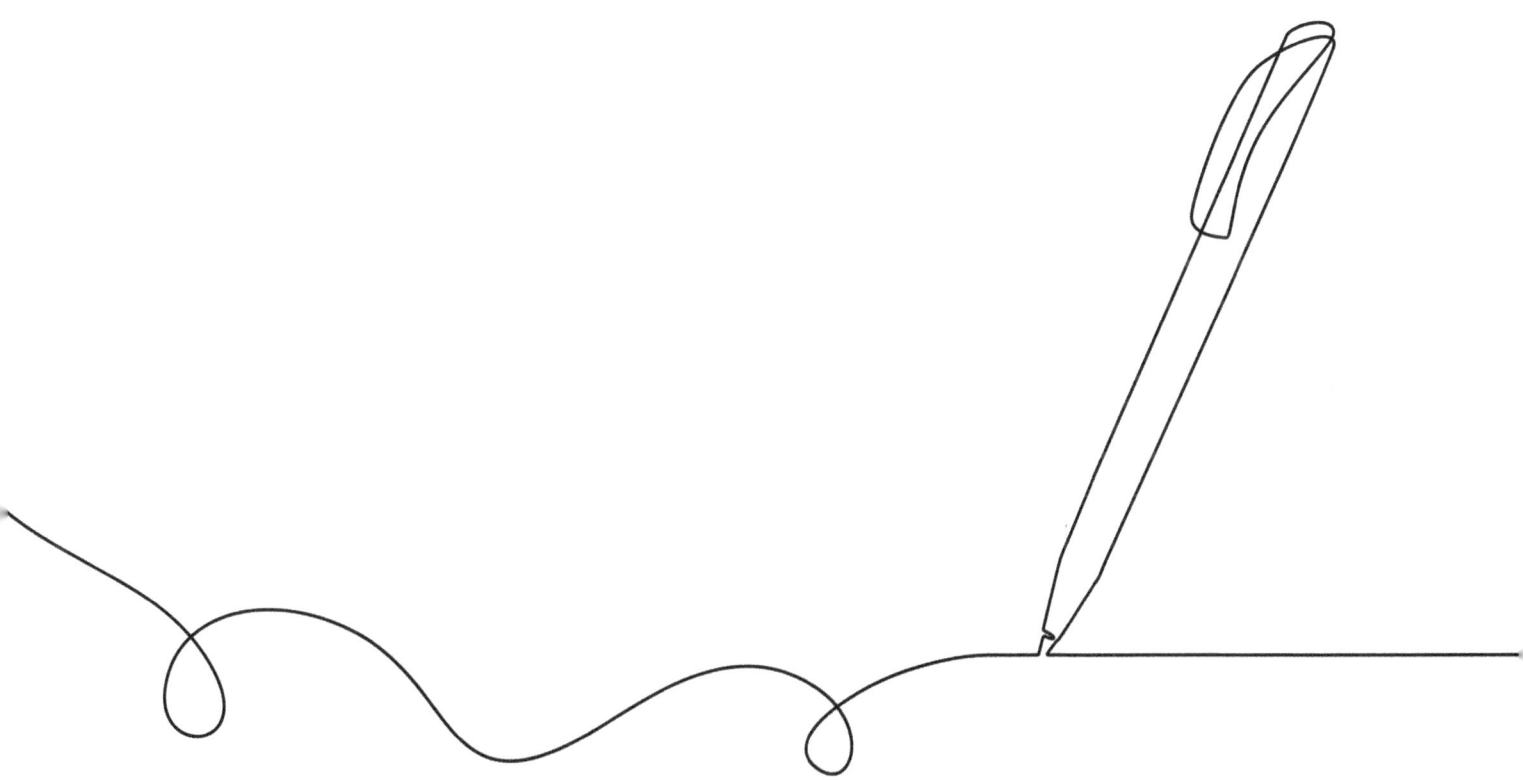

As hospitals grapple with shortages of nursing talent and aspire to advance healthcare in the 21st century, nurse leaders will be challenged to recruit and retain a culturally diverse workforce; that mirrors the populations we serve. This awakening to enhance diversity in nursing is not new to the profession; however, the need to successfully address this issue has never been greater.

The WANT is YOU, and the WHY is HEALTH EQUITY.

No matter the Age, Gender, Race, or Color... Go confidently towards your dreams, knowing your patients are waiting on **YOU.**

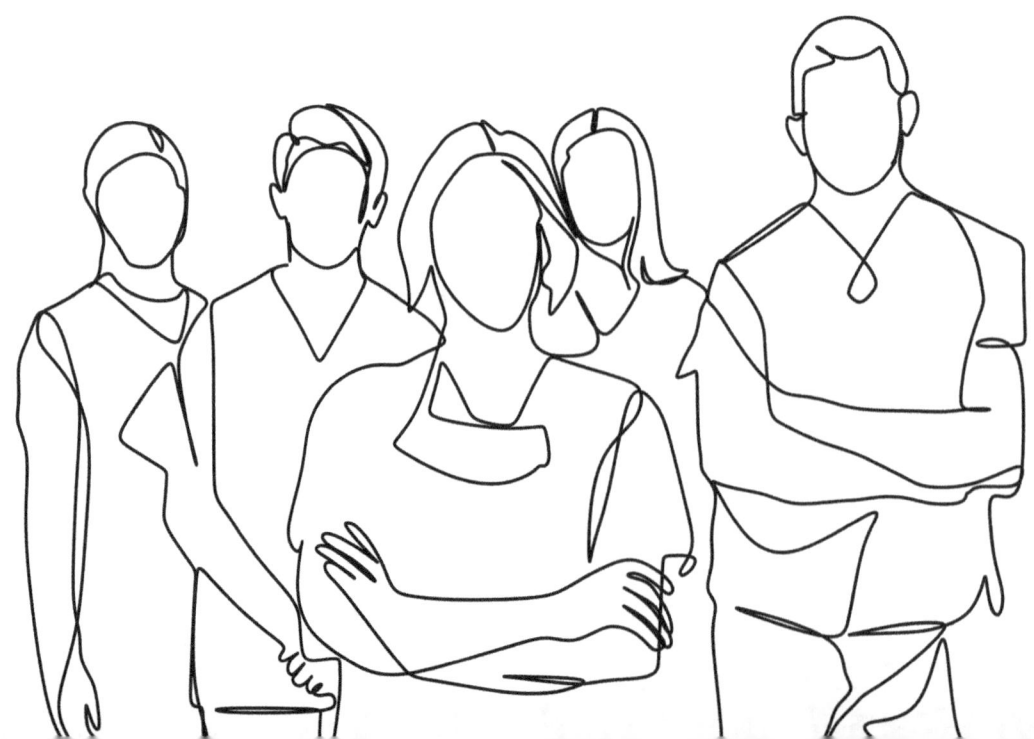

PUPIL2Peer
NURSING CONSULTING, LLC

BONUS

DIVERSITY
SPOTLIGHT

"We will not march back to what was. We move to what shall be, a country that is bruised, but whole. Benevolent, but bold. Fierce and free."

–Amanda Gorman

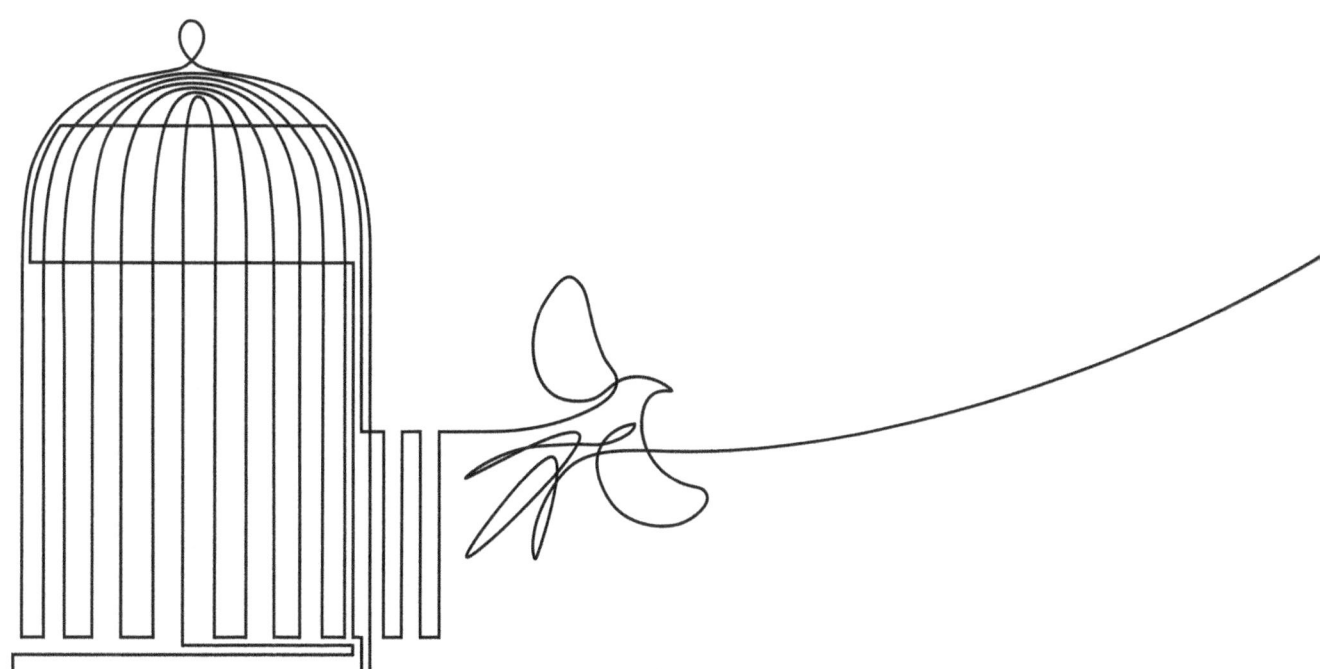

HISTORICALLY BLACK COLLEGE UNIVERSITIES

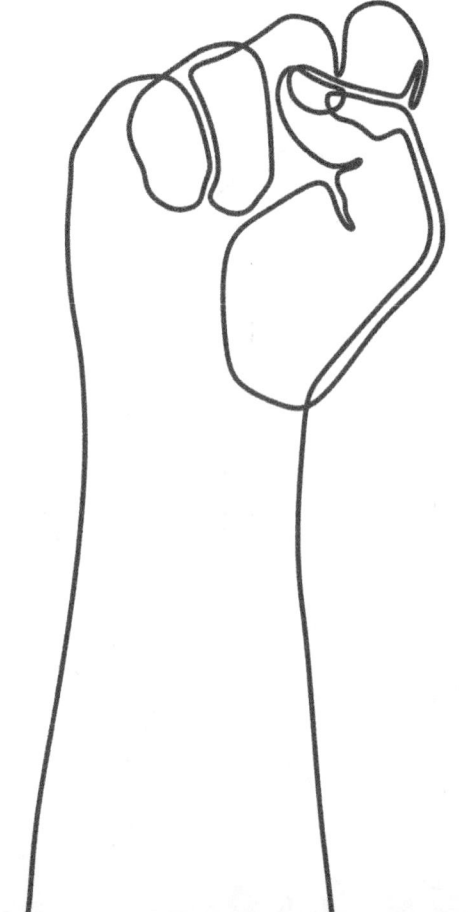

NATIONALLY ACCREDITED PROGRAMS

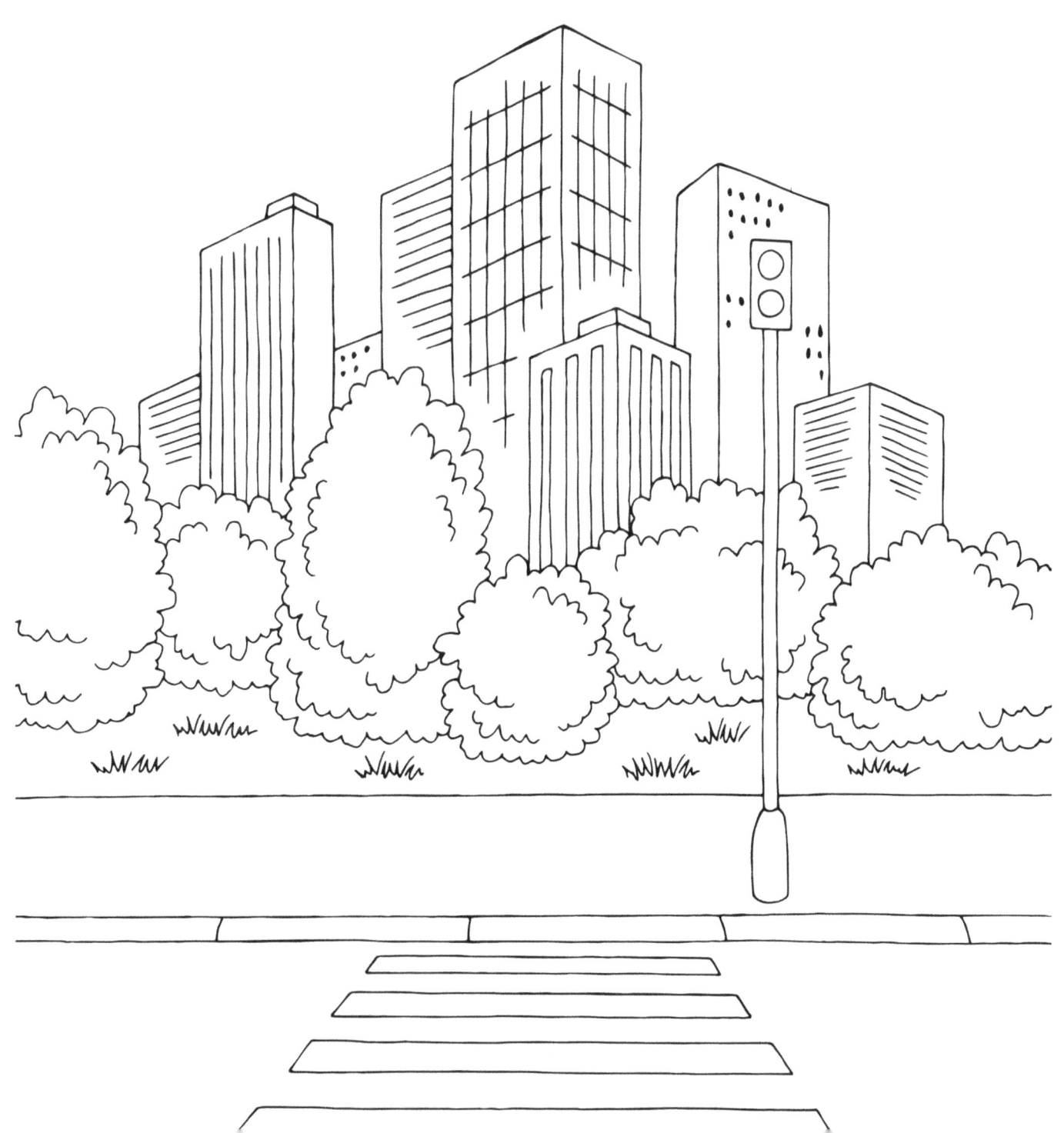

School	Location	Programs Offered
Albany State University	Albany, GA	Traditional, Evening, and Hybrid ASN Paramedic-to-RN LPN-to-RN Entry-Level BSN Accelerated BSN RN-to-BSN Master's
Alcorn State University	Lorman, MS	ASN LPN-to-ASN Entry-Level BSN RN-to-BSN Master's DNP
Bethune-Cookman University	Daytona Beach, FL	Entry-Level BSN
Bowie State University	Bowie, MD	Entry-Level BSN Master's Post Master's Certificate
Claflin University	Orangeburg, SC	RN-to-BSN Master's

School	Location	Programs Offered
Coppin State University	Baltimore, MD	Entry-Level BSN RN-to-BSN Accelerated BSN Master's DNP BSN-to-DNP Post Master's Certificate
Delaware State University	Dover, DE	Entry-Level BSN Master's
Dillard University	New Orleans, LA	Entry-Level BSN LPN-to-BSN RN-to-BSN
Fayetteville State University	Fayetteville, NC	Entry-Level BSN RN-to-BSN Master's
Florida Agricultural and Mechanical University	Tallahassee, FL	Entry-Level BSN RN-to-BSN Fast track RN-BSN Master's Post Master's Certificate
Grambling State University	Grambling, LA	Entry-Level BSN RN-to-BSN Master's Post Master's Certificate

School	Location	Programs Offered
Hampton University	Hampton, VA	Entry-Level BSN
		LPN-to-BSN
		PhD
		RN-to-BSN
		RN-to-MSN
		Master's
Howard University	Washington, DC	Entry-Level BSN
		LPN-to-BSN
		RN-to-BSN
		Master's
Kentucky State University	Frankfort, KY	ASN
		Entry-Level BSN
		RN-to-BSN
		DNP
Langston University	Langston, OK	Entry-Level BSN
		LPN-to-RN
		RN-to-BSN
Lincoln University	Jefferson City, MO	ASN
		Entry-Level BSN
		RN-to-BSN
Morgan State University	Baltimore, MD	Entry-Level BSN
		Master's
		PhD

School	Location	Programs Offered
Norfolk State University	Norfolk, VA	Entry-Level BSN RN-to-BSN
North Carolina A & T State University	Greensboro, NC	Accelerated BSN Entry-Level BSN RN-to-BSN RN-to-BSN (part-time)
North Carolina Central University	Durham, North Carolina	Accelerated BSN Entry-Level BSN RN-to-BSN Veteran-to-BSN
Oakwood University	Huntsville, AL	Entry-Level BSN RN-to-BSN
Prairie View A & M University	Houston, TX	Entry-Level BSN LPN-to-BSN RN-to-BSN Master's MSN-to-DNP
Southern University and A & M College	Baton Rouge, LA	Entry-Level BSN Master's DNP Ph.D.

School	Location	Programs Offered
Tennessee State University	Nashville, TN	Entry-Level BSN RN-to-BSN Master's Post Master's certificate
Tuskegee University	Tuskegee, AL	Entry-Level BSN RN-t- BSN
University of Arkansas at Pine Bluff	Pine Bluff, AR	Entry-Level BSN RN-to-BSN
University of the Virgin Islands	Charlotte Amalie, USVI	Entry-Level BSN
Virginia State University	Petersburg, VA	RN-to-BSN
West Virginia State University	Institute, WV	Entry-Level BSN
Winston – Salem State University	Winston – Salem, NC	Accelerated BSN Master's Entry-Level BSN LPN-to-BSN Paramedic-to-RN RN-to-BSN

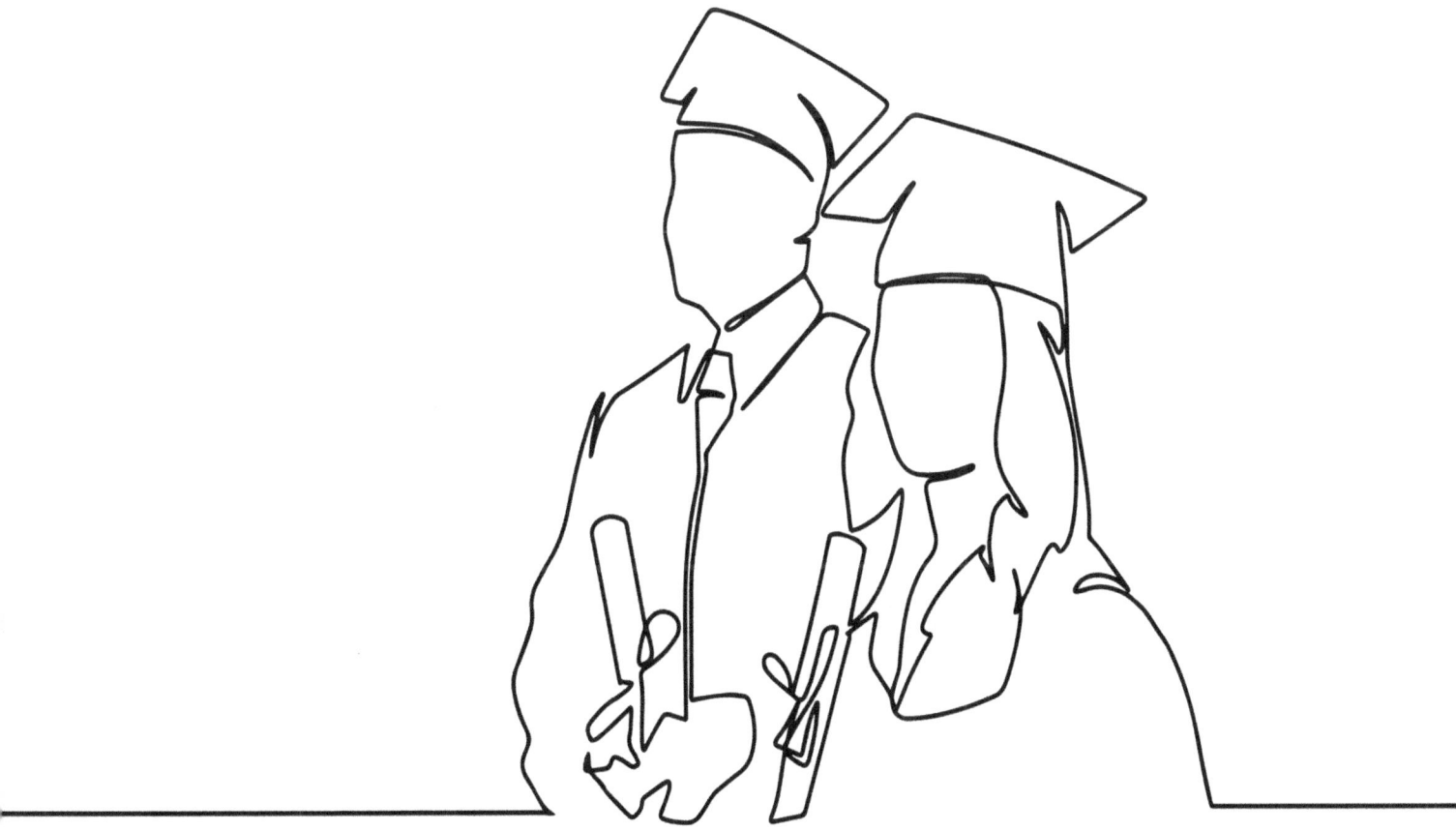

SCHOOLS:

TASKS TO DO:

NOTES:

SCHOOLS:

TASKS TO DO:

NOTES:

APPENDIX

RESOURCES

AACN Fact Sheet - Nursing Shortage. https://www.aacnnursing.org/News-Information/Fact-Sheets/Nursing-Shortage

AACN Nursing Education Programs. https://www.aacnnursing.org/Nursing-Education

ABSN Degree | Johnson & Johnson Nursing. https://nursing.jnj.com/nursing-degrees/accelerated-bachelors/

A Career in Nursing - NursingCAS. https://nursingcas.org/a-career-in-nursing/

ADN Nursing | Johnson & Johnson Nursing. https://nursing.jnj.com/nursing-degrees/associates/

BSN Degree | Johnson & Johnson Nursing. https://nursing.jnj.com/nursing-degrees/bachelors/

College Navigator | National Center for Education Statistics. https://nces.ed.gov/collegenavigator/

Financial Aid & Scholarships. https://www.aacnnursing.org/Students/Financial-Aid

How to Apply to Nursing School | Johnson & Johnson Nursing. https://nursing.jnj.com/applying-to-nursing-school

How to Apply - NursingCAS. https://nursingcas.org/how-to-apply/

Increasing Racial/Ethnic Diversity in Nursing to Reduce Health https://www.jstor.org/stable/23646785

National Nursing Workforce Study | NCSBN. https://www.ncsbn.org/cps/rde/xchg/SID-AE7346D2-6CCA17EC/ncsbn2018/hs.xsl/workforce.htm

Nursing Degrees and Programs | Johnson & Johnson Nursing. https://nursing.jnj.com/nursing-degrees

Nursing Degrees and Programs | Johnson & Johnson Nursing. https://nursing.jnj.com/nursing-degrees

Summary - The National Academies Press. https://nap.nationalacademies.org/read/25982/chapter/2

Ward-Smith, P. (2016). Evidence-Based Nursing: When the Evidence Is Fraudulent. Urologic Nursing, 36(2), 98.

What's the Deal with Accreditation? - NursingCAS. https://nursingcas.org/whats-the-deal-with-accreditation/

Why Nursing School Accreditation Matters | All Nursing Schools. https://www.allnursingschools.com/how-to-get-into-nursing-school/school-accreditation/

Work as a Nurse in the United States | Johnson & Johnson Nursing. https://nursing.jnj.com/work-in-the-united-states/

THE MEANING OF LIFE IS TO FIND YOUR GIFT. THE PURPOSE OF LIFE IS TO GIVE IT AWAY."

– PABLO PICASSO.

jrb

M B A - H C M , B S N , R N , O C N